T0130091

BONEHEAD
ELECTROCARDIOGRAPHY

BONEHEAD
ELECTROCARDIOGRAPHY

The Easiest and Best Way to Learn How to
Read Electrocardiograms—No Bones about It!

JOHN R. HICKS; FLOYD W. BURKE

Text Contribution: Hart Parker, MD
Technical Assistance: Demetra Caldera
Editorial Assistance: Henry Price, PhD
Cover Art: Gracie E. Hicks

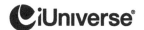

BONEHEAD ELECTROCARDIOGRAPHY
THE EASIEST AND BEST WAY TO LEARN HOW TO READ
ELECTROCARDIOGRAMS—NO BONES ABOUT IT!

iUniverse books may be ordered through booksellers or by contacting:

iUniverse
1663 Liberty Drive
Bloomington, IN 47403
www.iuniverse.com
1-800-Authors (1-800-288-4677)

Because of the dynamic nature of the Internet, any web addresses or links contained in this book may have changed since publication and may no longer be valid. The views expressed in this work are solely those of the author and do not necessarily reflect the views of the publisher, and the publisher hereby disclaims any responsibility for them.

Any people depicted in stock imagery provided by Thinkstock are models, and such images are being used for illustrative purposes only.

Certain stock imagery © Thinkstock.

ISBN: 978-1-4759-3667-4 (sc)
ISBN: 978-1-4759-3668-1 (hc)
ISBN: 978-1-4759-3669-8 (e)

Library of Congress Control Number: 2013910791

Print information available on the last page.

iUniverse rev. date: 01/11/2017

EKG COMMANDMENTS

As stated by Dr. William P. Nelson, our Division Chief, mentor, friend, respected electrocardiographer, gifted bedside clinician, and distinguished cardiologist.

I
Part A: Thou shall not overinterpret the EKG.
Part B: Thou shall not underinterpret the EKG.

II
Beware of the mischievous EKG machine or, in these more advanced times, the computer. Don't even think of allowing the computer to interpret the EKG for you. If you do, do so at your own peril, as often the computer interpretation is false.

III
Beware of the treacherous technician or the grubby medical student! They mean no harm, but they can inadvertently misplace leads or improperly adjust settings on the machine, resulting in the creation of faulty data.

IV
Thou shall not attempt to interpret an EKG without looking at the patient's prior tracings—if you can get your hands on one. Looking at an old EKG will make your interpretation of the new one easier and more likely accurate.

V
Be cautious of the pernicious patient. That means to be cautious of artifacts that might appear on the EKG as a result of the patient hiccoughing, coughing, or shaking. These movements can inadvertently affect the appearance of the EKG and cause artifacts that might erroneously be interpreted as abnormalities that don't really exist.

CONTENTS

TABLE OF ABBREVIATIONS

ASH	asymmetric septal hypertophy
AV	atrioventricular
HOCM	hypertrophic obstructive cardiomyopathy
I.D.	intrinsicoid deflection
IHSS	idiopathic hypertrophic subaortic stenosis
JVD	jugular venous distention
LAE	left atrial enlargement
LAFB	left anterior fascicular block
LBBB	left bundle branch block
LPFB	left posterior fascicular block
LVE	left ventricular enlargement
LVH	left ventricular hypertrophy
MI	myocardial infarction
PAC	premature atrial contraction
PAT	paroxysmal atrial tachycardia
PMT	pacemaker mediated tachycardia
PR	PR interval
PVARP	post-ventricular atrial refractory period
PVC	premature ventricular contraction
RAE	right atrial enlargement
RBBB	right bundle branch block
RVE	right ventricular enlargement
RVH	right ventricular hypertrophy
SA	sinoatrial
SLE	systemic lupus erythematosus
SVT	supraventricular tachycardia
VPB	ventricular premature beats
WPW	Wolff-Parkinson-White (syndrome)

FOREWORD

The field of cardiology has seen the development of a remarkable number of sophisticated laboratory tests to evaluate all of the aspects of the heart in its healthy and diseased state. Electrophysiological studies, nuclear exercise testing, CT scans and PET scans to mention a few.

But since the time of Einthoven and his string galvanometer (1901 and a Nobel Peace Prize In Medicine in 1924) to the standard electrocardiogram machine of today, the twelve lead electrocardiogram, after a competent history and physical examination, remains the primary diagnostic tool in the evaluation of a patient's cardiovascular status. In the office, in the emergency room, in the EMS vehicle on the way to the hospital, interpretation of "all those squiggly lines" (as described by a radiology associate of mine) is critical to patient management.

Not surprisingly, therefore, literally hundreds of textbooks of all sizes and shapes have been written about the topic over the years. I still have my copy of *A Primer of Electrocardiography (1949)* by George Burch and Travis Winsor which cites material from Professor Richard Ashman, my old teacher of physiology at Louisiana State University, and is remarkably accurate in its content. Some of the many texts are highly technical and probe the electrophysiological basis for the tracings. Others, some with titles almost as "cute" as Bonehead Electrocardiography, present material at varying levels of sophistication.

Why then another textbook as is being offered by Drs. Burke and Hicks? Part of the answer lies in the intent of the authors, both of whom are former students of mine and both of whom are outstanding practitioners and teachers of cardiology. The latter appellation is key. Teachers! Theirs is a book which *teaches* about electrocardiography.

I have always maintained that there are three basic components of effective teaching.

First, the teacher must have a deep understanding of his material. The authors have demonstrated that aspect of teaching both in their accomplishments in the field and have in turn learned the fundamentals from a superb teacher of electrocardiography, William P. Nelson, MD, himself a true master of the subject.

Next, the teacher must be able to adapt his ability to present material to the level of sophistication of the intended audience. Telling what a P wave represents is said differently to a second year medical student than it is to a third year cardiology fellow and must be told at a different level of sophistication. The authors clearly understand that point and go about doing it effectively in this book. Finally, and most importantly, in my opinion, is the compelling, burning desire of the teacher to see to it that the student "really gets it." That beautiful "aha" moment, when the teacher knows that he has completed the transaction and that the communication system has actually worked. To appreciate the fact that the authors feel this and believe in this goal, read, as they implore you to, the preface to the text in detail. You can actually feel them there, talking to you and making sure that each step of the presentation makes sense.

There are several innovative ideas in the book, including the use of a rat model to explain electrical axis (after all, the lab rat has been used for research and teaching since time immemorial in medicine.) And they are concerned that the user begin with very basic concepts and progress gradually and confidently to a full understanding. This book will not be of interest to those highly skilled in the field of cardiology. But for medical students, residents, especially Medical Residents, practicing Internists and Family Physicians, ER physicians and Emergency Medical Technicians, this is a splendid and painless way to develop competence in the field. And for those who teach the subject to those students, the text will be of exceptional help.

Burke and Hicks have put together a lighthearted but serious and effective presentation of an important topic in the field of cardiology, a worthy addition, and have also enlarged upon the English vocabulary by expanding the definition of the term *Bonehead*. Reading and studying this new textbook will be rewarding in terms of the learning process for electrocardiography itself and will demonstrate why competent teachers are so important to the learning process in general. This is not just another textbook in the field; it is a tutorial in the classic sense of the term. The authors are there all the time, side by side with you, encouraging, stimulating, challenging and sharing. This is pedagogy at its very best.

O'Neill Barrett, Jr., MD
Distinguished Professor and Chairman Emeritus

PREFACE

Normally, we wouldn't ask anyone to endure actually reading the preface of any book, not even this one. But don't turn the page just yet! By investing the time and energy necessary to read the entire preface, you will be able to take full advantage of what follows. It's important to teach you right away that efficiency follows form.

So, you have come to the worrisome conclusion that you have to acquire some knowledge in order to interpret EKGs properly. There is no way around this, and you are searching for your best option to complete this onerous task. It turns out your discovery of *Bonehead Electrocardiography* is more fortuitous than you imagined. Because we have your attention for only a second before you instinctively skip to the first chapter, you need to understand a few things: (1) This book is like no other, anywhere! (2) The authors are "Boneheads" and are not ashamed to admit it. (3) Boneheads are not stupid; rather, they are smart and remarkably discriminating. (4) Boneheads have an enormous affection for levity, particularly when learning a difficult subject. (5) Boneheads can master any subject quickly and joyfully, but only when taught in a nontraditional and efficient way.

Now take a simple test for us to see whether this book is right for you. Be honest with yourself. Can you read books like Tolstoy's *Anna Karenina* in a weekend? If you can, then stop right here and don't buy this book—you are not a Bonehead! Go spend your hard-earned money on something else. If you sometimes have difficulty remembering your phone number, then our book will benefit you.

As an aspiring medical professional of almost any kind—whether you want to become, or are a nurse, doctor, physician's assistant, paramedic, or even an EKG monitor technician—you can count on having to demonstrate your ability to make accurate judgments about

EKGs and cardiac rhythm strips. We hope this book makes your job of learning how to read EKGs easy and entertaining.

You might be wondering how a book with *Bonehead* in the title could possibly be worth your time and money. If we had set out to impress you with our intellect, the title would read something like *Higher Intellectual Analysis of the Summation of Electrical Vectors Resulting from Action Potential Waves during Cardiac Synchronous Depolarization*. Nice name, but who in their right mind would buy and actually read such a book?

We need to expound a little more about what being a Bonehead truly means. First, although the term may superficially seem like an insult, it is not. In fact, many famous people were Boneheads—we suspect if you analyzed many highly successful people in the world, you would find that most of them had Bonehead traits. The first attribute of a bono fide Bonehead is the presence of an impressively poor short-term memory. It is also imperative to have difficulty understanding complex explanations to simple problems. Have you ever heard of the "Law of Parsimony" or Occam's Razor? It states that when something is complex and hard to understand, the simplest explanation is most likely correct. Boneheads employ the rule of parsimony as often as possible. They like complex subjects broken down into easy-to-digest fragments so that they make sense.

It's amazing how teachers violate the rule of parsimony in the classroom. They make the simplest of problems appear so complicated that even the sharpest minds have difficulty understanding them. This approach to teaching is the "sleight of hand" technique many educators use to distance themselves from their students. Although Boneheads have short attention spans, they are smart and quick to recognize ineffective old-school educators. Then they either lose interest entirely or search elsewhere for explanations.

We all know that in a course of study, you must ultimately prove your knowledge by passing an exam. Students have devised all sorts of strategies to prepare for tests. When some students prepare to take a test, they invest all their time and energy into memorizing as much as they possibly can. Then, on test day, they hope they are lucid enough to regurgitate most of what they have "learned." This really isn't learning at all. It's a waste of time. If you can't recall something a month from the time you learned it, did you really learn it in the first place? The "memorize and forget" approach to test-taking might help you pass tomorrow's exam, but it is not the best strategy for long-term, fund-of-knowledge building that you can put to practical use months and years from now.

The knowledge you need to be an expert on anything has to be deeply ingrained in your mind. It must be "inculcated" to be intimately understood—it has to become a part of you. If something you are attempting to accomplish makes no sense to do in the long term, it makes even less sense to do it in the short term. Think about it!

Boneheads abhor rote memory work but are excellent at the unique human quality of deductive reasoning, an invaluable talent not equally distributed in the population, by the way. This is important, because Boneheads typically struggle to recall tangential and unconnected facts. Facts that have no real use in day-to-day life are of little use anyway, so why bother memorizing them?

Now let's look more closely at the Bonehead approach to education as it pertains to EKGs.

There are several ways to go about teaching students how to interpret EKGs. One approach is to focus on EKG pattern memorization. Could you memorize a thousand or more patterns? We didn't think so, because that would be a difficult undertaking for even the brightest of the bright. Plus, it's not practical. The pattern memorization approach requires students to learn and remember what the EKG should normally look like in all twelve leads. It also requires that the student memorize all the combinations and permutations of all the pathological or disease situations that can occur in the heart. Then they must know how each of those diseases affects the appearance of those twelve leads. We suppose it would be possible for a person with a photographic memory to accomplish this, but clearly there is a better way for those of us who are less fortunate.

A better way to learn how to read EKGs is to understand how and why the EKG appears as it does in the first place. That is what *Bonehead Electrocardiography* is predicated on. This eliminates the need for unreliable rote memorization. However, acquiring this understanding is no easy task. **Teaching you to understand the EKG is our challenge, and our passion.** If we fail this, you have learned nothing, and you will fall deep into Bonehead Depression. We don't want that!

As Boneheads ourselves, we feel qualified to help you learn how to accurately read most EKGs. The process of learning won't be painless, but the rewards will be well worth the effort. If you stick with our method of teaching, which we call the Bonehead Method, you will be the envy of all of your colleagues.

Interpreting EKGs is not just to impress teachers; it is potentially serious business. If you are an aspiring doctor, you must possess a great deal of knowledge regarding EKG interpretation. If you are a medical student, you will undoubtedly find it necessary to moonlight one day in an emergency room somewhere to help ease your financial strain. Did you know you can make a fortune working the night shift in an ER? If you choose to moonlight, then you can count on a nurse or the new, young, non-Bonehead-trained doctor, approaching you with an EKG from a patient with chest pain. This usually occurs right after you have gone to sleep. Naturally, the nurse will eagerly anticipate your astute and well-considered analysis of the situation. "WHAT NOW, DOCTOR?" To respond correctly, you must be able to accurately interpret the EKG. At three o'clock in the morning with your mind in a fog, it will be difficult, if not impossible, to remember that ST-segment elevation in leads II, III, and AVF indicates an acute inferior wall myocardial infarction (heart attack). After reading this book, however, you will know that intuitively. Imagine, you don't have to rely solely on that memory of yours in this life-threatening situation. That's the sort of intellect you really want.

In this book, we have included many examples and case scenarios that will help you attach what you are learning to something real. This will help you as you try to remember what's important.

There are many EKG text books available, so why should you believe ours is the best? Because most books on EKG interpretation are confusing, won't hold your attention, and are simply unreadable.

As you read this book, you'll quickly start to understand the EKG. You'll be surprised at how easily you recall the facts you have learned. Easy recall is what we are after. And that's not all. As a bonus, we have included several clinical pearls throughout the book not only to make it a more interesting read but to broaden your fund of knowledge about diseases, which will help to integrate what you're learning and make it last.

Because we put substance before form, some of the pictures,

examples, and images as drawn aren't intended to be exact renditions of actual human anatomy and physiology. They are, however, good and useful estimations thereof. This paradigm of using imagery makes it easier to teach you what you need to know to read most EKGs.

A word or two about references and bibliography—basically, there aren't any. Certainly, we used references and borrowed some ideas from authors of the textbooks we have read over the years, and we acknowledge these authors where appropriate to avoid going to jail for plagiarism. Much of the information presented, however, is an amalgamation of our unique understanding of cardiac physiology and medicine that sprang out of our experience over the years. As a result, it's difficult, if not impossible, to attribute any single author or reference any one textbook for factual information presented herein. We ask that you accept it as common knowledge to a practicing cardiologist.

Dr. William Nelson, our mentor and former Director of the Cardiology Fellowship at the University of South Carolina School of Medicine in Columbia (where we trained), provided numerous handouts that helped formulate our unique understanding of EKGs and how to read them. Unfortunately, Dr. Nelson never revealed his sources on some of the cartoons he used to teach us. As a result, you might see some pictures in our text that bear a resemblance to those in other publications. Where no specific reference is mentioned, it's because we don't have one, not because we didn't want to give due credit. Lastly, the "rat model" technique on teaching how to calculate the electrical axis is a unique and novel approach that had its genesis at one o'clock in the morning at a desk in an apartment at 90 Radcliffe Street in Charleston, South Carolina, while one of the authors (JH) was a lowly Bonehead medical student, like many of you reading this book right now!

To make certain that everyone reading the book has a fair start, we begin by assuming that all readers know absolutely nothing about EKGs. This will alleviate any worry you have that you will be lost in the beginning. Now on to chapter 1. Let's learn some EKG!

John R. Hicks, MD
Floyd W. Burke, MD

CHAPTER 1: THE BONEHEAD BASICS

WARNING: IF YOU DID NOT READ THE PREFACE, YOU REALLY ARE A BONEHEAD! GO BACK AND READ IT NOW!

Uh-oh! You have concluded that there is no escaping the fact that you will have to be able to interpret EKGs. You can't fake your way through this one—no matter how hard you try or how smart you think you are. It is as compulsory to your career as a triple toe loop is to a competitive figure skater. Where are you going to start? How could you possibly learn what all those squiggly lines mean on that funny-looking graph paper? You might even entertain thoughts of making a quick career change when faced with the reality of being required to interpret EKGs. Surely becoming a rocket scientist would be easier than what you are trying to accomplish. Fortunately, we're here to help you devise a strategy to see you through the process of becoming a first-rate EKG interpreter.

At first glance, EKG interpretation appears to be an overwhelming, not to mention complicated undertaking. The learning process can be almost painless and interesting—but only for those who indulge us. We provide the map, the strategy, and the process. You need to supply the time, energy, and enthusiasm (and maybe a little trust that we know what we're talking about), and you will achieve the results you desperately need.

The information and teaching techniques in this book will prove a powerful tool to medical students, interns, residents, physician's assistants, nurses, EMTs, and other paramedical professionals as they begin the career-long journey to EKG reading competency. It does take time and effort to become a proficient EKG reader, and the time invested in mastering this subject could pay huge dividends. You just might save someone's life someday.

We prefer that you start by reading the book from beginning to end—don't skip around. You will learn much faster this way, because each concept presented is carefully structured and builds on the one preceding it. Please take care to learn and understand each topic before going to the next paragraph. So avoid any temptation to "skim and resume." After completing the entire book, you can then refer back to sections as needed. The chapters have been set up the way they are so that even someone who knows nothing about EKGs can learn. We could teach a high schooler working as a bag boy at the grocery store if he took a notion to read this book in earnest.

The order of presentation is self-evident, so we won't repeat it here. We believe it best to start with what the EKG is supposed to do—meaning, its job. Then, we teach you how the EKG is designed to accomplish that job. In nature, design reflects purpose and vice versa. Why should the EKG be any different?

The EKG, Its Purpose and Design

The heart is unique in that is the only organ in the body that has an electrical charge in the resting state (except the brain). When an object is charged, it is said to be **polarized**. That is what polarized means—electrically charged. Something must be polarized before it can **depolarize**. The heart just sits there polarized and waits to depolarize, or release its charge, as it goes about its work, which is to squeeze the blood out to the body. The heart depends on a signal to tell it to mechanically contract, or beat. This signal to contract is the process of depolarization of the polarized cell membranes within the heart. Once the heart has depolarized and contraction has occurred, it must repolarize so the process can repeat itself. Without the seesaw effect of cardiac polarization, depolarization, and repolarization, there would be no heartbeat, no EKG machine, no human life, and you wouldn't be sitting there reading this book, and we wouldn't have written it. That's pretty certain.

The EKG is designed to record the electrical activity of the heart as it beats. It then leaves a permanent recording of the multiple depolarization and repolarization events that occur with every beat of the heart.

In order to be useful to the interpreter, the EKG must reveal important clinical information that a doctor can use to diagnose what's wrong with a patient. To accomplish its job completely, the EKG must be able to observe the heart from as many locations as possible. It can't look just at the back or front. No, it has a much larger task. It has to record information from the front, back, top, bottom, and sides. After the EKG machine records the information, it has to present it to the interpreter in a consistent and recognizable format. The interpreter, we hope, will learn a little something about the patient who had the EKG performed. This information might be critical in determining if a heart issue is contributing to the patient's ailment.

In order to accomplish this task of assessing the heart's electrical activity in its entirety, a **twelve-lead system** has been devised. The system didn't have to have twelve leads. It could have been more or less, but those who discovered and developed the EKG settled on twelve leads, so twelve it is. Each lead of the twelve-lead system has a name (or label if you prefer) and a job. The job of each lead is to record the electrical activity of the heart as it sees it. Obviously, an individual lead can see only a small area of the heart, so this is why it takes twelve leads to complete the survey. Simple enough so far!

For a twelve-lead EKG system to record all areas of the heart, the leads must view the heart from two different planes. These planes are orthogonal to each other, which means at right angles. These ninety-degree opposing planes of view are situated in front of the patient. One plane looks straight through toward the back of the patient, and the other is in front, looking across the patient from side to side. These arrangements of two distinct planes of view are appropriately named the **frontal** and the **horizontal** planes. Don't panic—pictures will follow to help you visualize this.

One plane views the front surface of the patient, while the other looks directly through the patient from front to back. The horizontal plane really should have been named the "front to back" plane, while the frontal plane should have been named the "front surface only head to toe" plane. Confused? Just wait! To help with the visual, think of a patient standing up. Now imagine the horizontal plane as cutting the patient in half through the waist. The horizontal plane is the cut surface of the two halves. Another analogy is that the horizontal plane looks at the rings of a chopped down tree, while the frontal plane sees only the bark. Got it? Again, we have a picture a few paragraphs below to help.

The twelve-lead EKG is subdivided into two halves, each consisting of two six-lead categories. Six of the twelve leads view the heart in the frontal plane. The remaining six leads view the heart in the horizontal plane. How convenient—we have two equally divided planes of view in this system. Hang in there. It gets a little more complicated, but not much.

The **limb leads** view the heart from the **frontal plane**. It is important to remember this, so we'll say it again: the limb leads view the heart in the frontal plane. That means these leads scan the heart's frontal surface (or the bark of the tree, already mentioned). Of course, there are six of these leads.

The **chest leads** (also called "V" leads) view the heart in the **horizontal plane**. To clarify, this means they see straight through the heart as if looking from front to back, or in cross-section, as though the patient had been sawed in half. These leads "see" the rings of the tree.

Again, it is critical to know that there are six limb leads and six chest leads. Remember that the terms chest leads and V leads are interchangeable. This multilead setup allows for maximal viewing of the heart by the EKG. Physiologic abnormalities of the heart will often, but not always, be revealed as electrical abnormalities recorded by the EKG. Again, we must have a full disclosure of all ongoing electrical cardiac events to diagnose problems. The twelve-lead system enables us to view almost all areas of the heart—although, as you will see later, one small segment of the heart remains elusive. See figures 1 and 2 to help you understand how the leads are arranged around the patient.

Figure 1. Leads and their location relative to the heart in the frontal plane. These are the limb leads. They scan or look at the heart in the frontal plane.

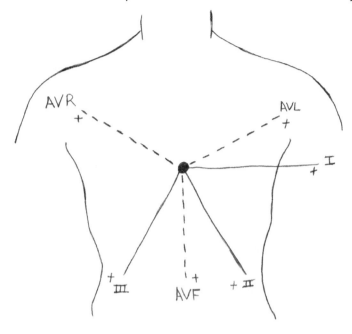

Figure 2. Leads and their location relative to the heart in the horizontal plane. These are the "V" leads. They are also called chest leads. They scan the heart in an anterior-posterior direction, or from front to back.

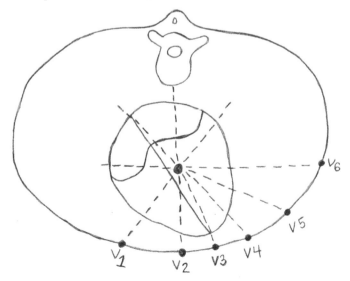

The Leads

The EKG consists of twelve leads arranged around the heart at different locations. As a result, each lead can see a different area of the myocardium (or heart muscle). Think of it as twelve sets of eyeballs located around and scanning the heart for any electrical activity. Each lead, or "eyeball," looks at a specific and fairly limited area of the heart.

Some of this is redundant, but Boneheads thrive on redundancy. The limb leads are comprised of the following: leads I, II, III, AVR, AVL, and AVF. They view the heart in the frontal plane. The precordial leads (or chest or V leads, whichever term you prefer) include leads V_1, V_2, V_3, V_4, V_5, and V_6. They look at the heart in the horizontal plane.

It might help you to ask an EKG technician to teach you how to place all ten EKG wires correctly on a patient having an EKG. That way, you will readily recognize a lead placement error should it occur. Although there are only ten wires, from these ten wires we can record twelve leads. Sound confusing? It will become clearer.

The EKG Paper

When looking at the paper on which the EKG is inscribed, note that it's divided into both **small** and **large** boxes. Time is measured on the X-axis, or horizontally across the paper. At a standard paper speed of 25 millimeters per second, each small box then represents 0.04 seconds, or 40 milliseconds of time, that is, when the paper is moving. Each large box then equates to 0.2 seconds, or 200 milliseconds. Note that there are five small boxes that make up one large box. Five large boxes make up a time interval of one second. Look at the EKG paper carefully and learn this now. You must know this to move forward.

On the Y-axis, or vertically up the paper, voltage is measured. It is standard that one large vertical box (consisting of again five small boxes) equals 0.5 millivolts of electrical activity sensed by the EKG lead doing the observing. EKGs sensing more massive amounts of myocardium depolarizing will record proportionally higher spikes. Smaller hearts generate less electrical energy, and the EKG reflects this by inscribing smaller spikes. That should make sense to you. The more electrical activity recorded, the taller the EKG spike will appear. The converse is true as well—just to make sure you got it. So the take-home message is that a small amount of myocardium depolarizing will result in the appearance of a small EKG spike, while large (or hypertrophied) hearts will generate large spikes. Understanding this will be helpful when determining the heart rate, measuring the duration of depolarization or repolarization, calculating intervals, or determining if the cardiac heart chamber is enlarged. Of course, we will explain all this in more detail as we go along. By design, the EKG is presented in the format in figure 3 so that the leads can be properly ascribed to their position on the EKG paper.

Figure 3. Normal EKG layout: please notice where the limb and chest leads are located on the EKG printout. They are clearly labeled on the EKG paper. There can be some variation from hospital to hospital, but this is usually how it is recorded. Note that the very bottom recording, or line of spikes, is just a continuous recording of the electrical activity as seen in a single lead—in this case, lead II.

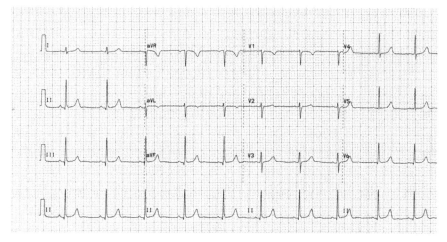

The EKG Electrical Spikes: P Waves, QRS, T Waves, and Everything Else

As you look at an EKG, you immediately notice several waves and spikes. All these waves and spikes that make up an EKG have names, which you'll need to know. While trying to learn how to read EKGs, your job will be easier if you question why the waves and spikes appear as they do in the first place. Once you understand this, you'll be better able to read EKGs. It's our ambition to teach you exactly what the spikes and waves represent and what makes them appear the way that they do.

It'll all make sense to you soon, because the EKG really isn't that complicated. Its function is predicated on the fact that in order for the heart to beat, an electrical impulse, called an action potential, must occur. The EKG machine witnesses and records this electrical event. The machine inscribes what it sees on the EKG paper. Everyone's heart, as it contracts, leaves an "electrical trail" that is unique to it. A normal heart will leave a normal electrical trail, while an abnormal heart will leave a trail that is abnormal. The EKG machine simply records whatever electrical activity it observes while the heart is beating.

In order to interpret an EKG, you must understand that the morphology (shape or appearance) of the electrical spikes recorded on the EKG paper is determined by only three things.

First is the mass (or amount) of myocardium (again, heart muscle) depolarizing, which is reflected in the voltage recorded on the EKG paper and ultimately is the determining factor in how tall or short the EKG spikes are.

Second is the direction in which the electrical impulse is traveling relative to the location of the EKG lead recording it. This then determines the polarity of the EKG spike. By polarity we mean whether the EKG spike is upright or down-going. A down-going spike is also termed a **negative deflection**. Look at the above EKG and notice that some of the spikes go above the baseline and some below. Soon you will know why this is so. Not only will you know why, but you'll also be able to predict how the spikes are supposed to look. Each time an action potential occurs, the electrical energy will travel in a specific direction and for a finite amount of time. Not only that, but the voltage, or amount of energy generated by the heart, can be measured by the machine with each contraction of the heart. All these variables determine how the EKG ultimately looks.

The third thing is the length of time it takes the electrical impulse to travel from where it started to wherever it stops. Obviously, if the paper speed is set at a constant speed and doesn't change, then a narrow spike means the impulse travels quickly. A wide spike, on the other hand, indicates slow propagation of the electrical activity. The slower the impulse travels, the wider the spike will become.

The EKG is uniquely and specifically designed to follow certain rules. Let's review them. You must be familiar with these rules to understand how the EKG works. It is only by understanding how the machine works that you can think beyond rote memorization of EKG patterns.

The rules you need to know about how the EKG is designed to function are short and simple. By design, any given EKG lead must record an **upright** deflection when it sees an electrical impulse traveling **toward** it. If, on the other hand, this same lead sees an electrical impulse traveling **away** from it, a **negative** (or down-going) deflection must be recorded. Look again at the normal EKG example in figure 3. See the lead AVR, for instance, and notice that the large electrical spike goes down, or is negative.* Notice also, in contrast, that in AVF the spike (QRS again) is positive, or upright. Now, also understand that if a spike can go up or down, it can do both. A spike that is both up and down is called an **isoelectric** spike. An equal up and down spike occurs when an EKG lead witnesses an action potential traveling exactly **perpendicular** to its fixed location. Now, look at lead V_3 and see the isoelectric spike in figure 3. Reread this section if you have to. It is imperative that you understand this fully before moving forward.

It is important also to recognize that the magnitude (or height) of the deflection recorded on the EKG is a function of the amount of electrical activity generated by the depolarizing heart. The more heart that there is to depolarize, the more voltage will be generated. The increased voltage will result in a larger EKG spike. So a thickened heart, one with left ventricular hypertrophy, for instance, will naturally result in large spikes recorded on the EKG.

Let's now summarize some basics. Physiology, coupled with how the EKG is designed, dictates that a *large* mass of myocardium depolarizing *toward* a specific EKG electrode will cause a *large upright* deflection in that lead (you must understand this). A *small* mass of myocardium depolarizing *toward* an electrode causes a *small upright* deflection. A *large* mass of myocardium depolarizing *away* from an electrode causes

---

* Referred to as a "QRS" by convention and representing the majority of the heart depolarizing and contracting.

a *large negative,* or *down-going* deflection. A wave of electrical activity moving *perpendicular* to an electrode causes an *isoelectric* deflection. Remember that isoelectric means half up and half down.

See the illustration below and be sure you have a good grasp of these rules. Note that in the diagram, the electrical impulse starts on the left side of the paper and travels horizontally to the right side, where it completes its brief journey. This event is equivalent to one beat of the heart. We have drawn crude eyeballs to designate the locations of the four leads witnessing this hypothetical depolarizing event. Next to each eyeball, we have drawn what the QRS or EKG spike should look like. The eyeball will record the spike (or QRS) based on the rules we went over above. In the figure below, notice that the eyeball on the far left sees the wave of depolarization traveling directly away from it. Since the eyeball (or lead, if you prefer) on the far left sees the action potential traveling in a direction directly away from its vantage point, it must therefore record a negative deflection. You can deduce the rest. Take a break and think about all that you have learned. Visualize, visualize. That is the easiest way to learn this.

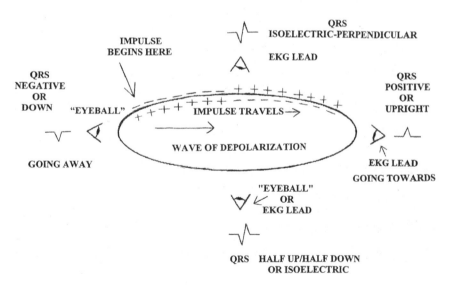

Now, let's look at the width of the EKG spike as opposed to its polarity (up or down) and overall size. The width, or duration, of the EKG spike is determined again by only two things. The first one is the paper speed (at a standardized 25 millimeters per second), which we don't have to concern ourselves with, because it shouldn't change. The second thing is the amount of time required for the electrical impulse to travel throughout the myocardium (heart muscle). Electrical impulses that follow the normal conduction pathways (including the AV node, right and left bundles and Purkinje fibers, all of which we will discuss later) result in EKG spikes that are narrow. They are narrow because they travel **fast**. Impulses that follow aberrant or abnormal pathways, or originate outside the usual electrical pathways, for that matter, are usually wide. The reason they are wide is that the specialized normal conduction tissue that the action potential is supposed to use conducts electricity rapidly, while myocardial cell-to-cell dissemination of electrical activity is comparatively slow. If the normal conduction sequence is not followed, then the only way for the action potential to spread is through the slower process of cell-to-cell electrical conduction. The heart is magnificently constructed to do its job efficiently and quickly. It takes advantage of specialized tissues that conduct electricity quickly when functioning normally. We will go over all the anatomy of the heart later, so don't get too hung up on the terms we just mentioned.

NOTE: Recall that when the heart muscle depolarizes, all areas of the heart are depolarizing virtually simultaneously. Not only do they depolarize at the same time, but they do so in different directions. The EKG records the sum total of all the depolarizations occurring at any given time. The aforementioned culminates in the EKG machine recording "waves" that represent a resultant electrical **vector**. Oh no! Vector! Bet you weren't expecting that word to crop up. Keep reading, and we will explain some more, but in a broad sense, think of a person being held by all four extremities and pulled hard in four different directions by four different people of varying sizes and strength. Where the person's belly button ends up when all the pulling is finished is the resultant vector.

If you have ever taken physics, you may recall that vectors have magnitude, direction, and sense. To illustrate this, consider the heart in figure 4 with the relatively small right ventricle depolarizing from the endocardium (inside) to the epicardium (outside). At the same time, the larger left ventricle depolarizes from the endocardium to the epicardium, but in a direction opposite that of the right ventricle. So, the right side of the heart is doing its thing while the left side does its thing. Look at figure 4 and visualize this now. Since the electrical events are going in opposite directions, the events would cancel each other out, except for the fact that the left side is much bigger. Because the left side is bigger, it generates more electricity, which will overshadow the events occurring on the right side. This results in the right ventricle contributing a small amount of electricity, pulling the resultant vector to the right, while the left ventricle contributes a large amount of electricity, pulling the vector to the left. The resultant vector is the sum of these two simultaneous forces in relation to their magnitudes and directions. The final vector points leftward and overshadows the right ventricular component. If the left and right sides of the heart were exactly the same size, then the fat arrow below would point straight down instead of being tilted to the left as it is drawn. The very small arrows illustrate the component parts that contribute to the final vector. It's very similar to an electrical tug-of-war. It will be important to understand and remember this concept later.

Figure 4. Normal cardiac depolarization.

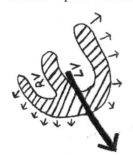

QRS AXIS OR MEAN RESULTANT VECTOR

Normal Sequence of Depolarization and Repolarization

In the normal heart, the electrical impulse originates in the **sinoatrial** (SA) node. This is located at the junction of the superior vena cava and right atrium. If you don't know, the superior vena cava is the large vein that drains all the blood out of the head and arms and empties it into the right atrium of the heart (which is the holding chamber for deoxygenated blood returning from the body) to prepare it for a trip to the lungs to pick up oxygen.

For those of you who know little about the anatomy of the heart, let us mention that the human heart has four chambers: two chambers on top and two on the bottom. It also has two chambers on the left and two on the right, as nature likes symmetry. The two upper chambers are called the right and left atria. The bottom chambers are the right and left ventricles. Think of the atria as blood collectors or depositories and the ventricles as strong pumpers. The right ventricle pumps blood to and through the lungs to load red blood cells with oxygen, and the left ventricle pumps recently oxygenated blood to the rest of the body, excluding the lungs.

From a functional perspective, the right atrium receives deoxygenated blood from the body that needs oxygen replenishment before returning to the body to deliver more. This oxygen-poor blood is stored for a brief period in the right atrium while it is collected. After a short interval, it then is dumped into the right ventricle. From there, it is subsequently pumped out to the lungs. In the lungs, the blood picks up oxygen and then travels to the left atrium via the pulmonary veins. Upon arrival to the left atrium, it is collected for a brief period and is then deposited into the left ventricle as a result of contraction of the left atrium. Now the real miracle of life and circulation begins to unfold. The left ventricle is a very powerful pump, thickly walled with amazing strength and ability. It is the left ventricle that has the responsibility to contract and propel the oxygen-rich blood to all the tissues of the body. Think about it for just a moment. This little pump is able to send blood through miles of arteries and capillaries with each single squeeze. It does this by creating enormous pressure in a closed system with only one way out. And that way is through the aortic valve (a one-way valve between the left ventricle and the aorta). The aorta is as big around as a standard hose pipe and many times as strong. The aorta then carries the blood to the many branch blood vessels that supply all the tissues of the body. The smaller vessels are called arteries and carry oxygenated blood. The blood returns to the heart after delivering the oxygen to the tissue in small flexible and thin tubes called veins. As the veins carry blood containing very little oxygen, they appear bluish-green, and the blood inside is a very dark red, as opposed to the blood in arteries, which is loaded with oxygen; this blood is bright red like a fire truck. So, if you ever have the occasion to stick a needle into a patient to get venous blood out to send to the lab and instead you see that the blood is bright red, you might want to reconsider where your needle is, pull it out quickly, and hold pressure on the spot for a few minutes. Also, blood in the arteries is under high pressure and will shoot halfway across a small room, whereas venous blood just trickles out.

In order for the right atrium to empty its contents into the right ventricle, it must physically contract. To do this, it needs an electrical signal. This signal begins in the sinoatrial (or SA for short) node. This is where atrial electrical activation begins for each heartbeat. The SA node is commonly referred to as the pacemaker of the heart. Just know that the electrical signal to cause a beat of the heart starts at the top right-hand corner of the upper half of the heart. Just after the SA node fires, it activates the right atrium through natural transmission of electrical activity downward from its origin. This right atrial activation then travels through "Bachmann's" bundle to fire the left atrium. So, in this paradigm, the right atrium fires (or depolarizes) just before the left atrium; and by just before, we mean fractions of a second before. This electrical event corresponds to contraction of the two atria which will generate what we call a **P wave** on the EKG.

The P wave (which is correlated with atrial depolarization and contraction) is the first electrical spike of a cardiac contraction cycle. Since the atria are relatively small, the P wave is small as well. There is no need for the atria to be large and muscular, because they only have to gently squeeze to send the blood a few centimeters. The atrial impulse after firing the upper half of the heart also travels inferiorly (or downward) to the **atrioventricular** (AV) node. The AV node is the only electrical connection between the upper and lower parts of the heart. The lower half of the heart, which again includes the right and left ventricles, can't contract unless they receive an electrical impulse from the atria above. This electrical impulse must travel through the AV node, because the upper half and the lower half of the heart are electrically insulated from each other, and the only way for the impulse to get down to the ventricles is the electrical pathway called the AV node. It gets to the AV node from the atria through internodal tracts that are built into the atria, but that's not important for you to remember right now. Once the impulse reaches the AV node, a physiologic delay occurs, allowing time for mechanical atrial contraction. This atrial contraction is important, because it forces blood into the ventricles below. It doesn't do any good to squeeze an empty lower half of the heart! After the brief delay to allow the lower ventricles to fill with blood, the impulse then travels further downward to and through the **bundle of His**. This is simply a short segment of specialized tissue at the tail end of the AV node that is capable of carrying electrical energy more quickly. From there, it travels to and through both the **left and right bundle branches** before it ultimately reaches the ventricles. It travels through these bundle branches virtually simultaneously. Both the left and right bundles are the "electrical highways" that carry electricity from the bundle of His the remainder of the way down to both muscular ventricles.

Just to make it a little more complicated, note that the left bundle is unique in that it has two branches, called **fascicles**. They are called the left anterior and left posterior fascicles. We usually just refer to the combination of both fascicles comprising the left bundle collectively as the left bundle branch. The electrical impulse isn't through yet. It then proceeds to the **Purkinje fibers**, where it can now activate the heart. These fibers are like little tentacles on the tips of each bundle branch. The Purkinje fibers activate the ventricles sequentially from the endocardial surface (inside) to the epicardial surface (outside). Figure 5 should make this clear. You should probably study this figure until you can draw it from memory. This is a flowchart detailing how one beat of the heart propagates. As you look at it, imagine the entire sequence, starting in the SA node and traveling over to the left side of the heart and down in a careful and organized sequence. Now study the picture! As drawn in the picture, imagine that a patient has been cut in half through the shoulders down to the feet and the heart got in the way, separating the front half of the heart from the back, and you are looking at the heart in the now halved patient staring at the back half of the remaining heart.

Figure 5. Sagittal section of the heart.

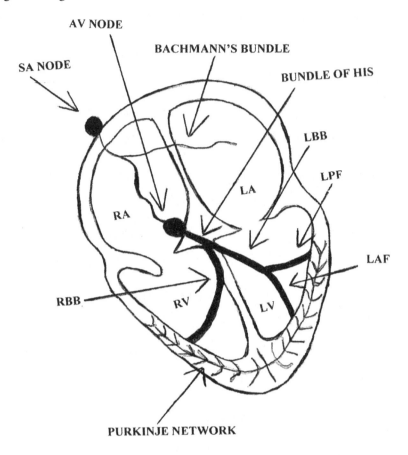

As a result of the anatomy and physiology of the heart's electrical conduction system, the myocardium normally depolarizes in a standard time and directional sequence, as illustrated in figure 6. Now, you are probably thinking, "Whoa, this is complicated!" You thought this was going to be easy. Well, it is, really. We don't want you to get bogged down in too many details. Just remember that the electrical impulse that begins a single contraction of the heart starts in the SA node at the top right corner of the right atrium. It then travels downward and to the left, activating both the right and left atria at just about the same time, but remember that the left atrium activates just slightly after the right atrium. The electrical stimulus then gets to the lower half of the heart, which is the right and left ventricles, through the electrical bridge called the AV node. Here, the impulse is delayed, allowing time for the contracting atria to fill the ventricles below. The muscular ventricles contract after receiving the impulse that traveled quickly through the bundle of His, both bundle branches, and finally the Purkinje fibers.

Ventricular contraction results in the occurrence of the relatively large QRS complex. Recall that the ventricles are big and muscular. You will recognize the QRS complex, because your eyes are drawn to it on the EKG, as it is the largest spike and hard to miss. The point is that the ventricles depolarize quickly and the QRS, which again correlates to ventricular depolarization, is therefore narrow. Note one more time that after the atria fire, there is a slight pause to let the lower half of the heart fill with blood; then, and only then, do the ventricles (the lower half two main pumping chambers of the heart) depolarize.

The process of ventricular depolarization has its own specific sequence of activation. It begins with ventricular septal activation. This is followed by depolarization of the right ventricle, and then the apex, or tip of the heart. The bulk of the left ventricle and finally the base of the heart depolarize last. For those of you who are interested, the base of the heart is the part of the heart that is anatomically close to the valves between the atria and ventricles. As such, the base is the highest part of the ventricles vertically. Also, note that the septal forces (the septum of the heart is the muscular tissue that separates the right and left ventricles) go from left to right. This is opposite of the remainder of the left ventricular myocardium, which go to the left side of the body. You do not have to memorize this right now; we just want you to have a general understanding.

The ultimate consequence of all these depolarizations is that the resultant electrical vector of left and right ventricular depolarization occurs quickly and normally points down and toward the patient's left side close to where the number 5 appears on the schematic as drawn in figure 6. This resultant vector we have been stressing is equivalent to the electrical axis of the heart. Don't worry, you will hear much more about that later.

If you have a hard time conceptualizing the electrical vector of ventricular depolarization, then we have an easier way to understand it. Think of a man wearing a necktie. Visualize the tie tilting and pointing toward the man's left hip; that is where the normal ventricular electrical axis is directed.

Figure 6. Normal cardiac depolarization.

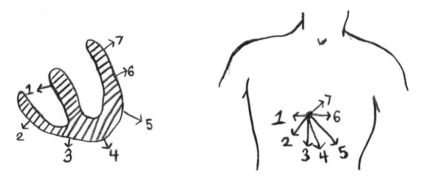

Now, why did we make you read all this detail? Sometimes, a block or failure of the electrical system occurs. This results in delayed activation of an area of the heart. This causes the EKG spike, or QRS, to become wider than usual, as illustrated in figure 7 with a **left bundle branch block** (LBBB) example.

Figure 7. LBBB: note the wide QRS as a result of a broken conduction system. The QRS is the larger of the spikes in each cardiac cycle, and it is wider than it should be.

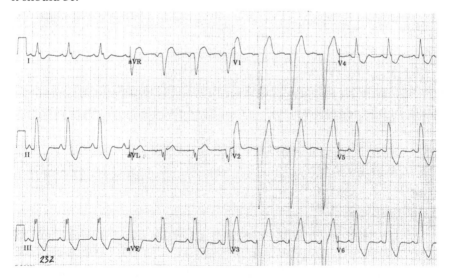

P Waves, Q Waves, T Waves, and QRS Complexes

By convention, the EKG consists of spikes or waves, each of which has an alphabetic designation. In a single cardiac cycle (that is, one heartbeat), the atria depolarize first. This event is seen as a spike, called a **P wave**. This is the first wave of a normal cardiac cycle seen on an EKG. Again, it marks atrial depolarization and is usually fairly short, small, and narrow. It is the smallest spike you will see, and as such it is easily recognized. This is followed by a physiologic delay (in the AV node), which is manifested as the **PR interval** (PR) on the EKG. It is the amount of time it takes the electrical impulse to travel from the atria to the ventricle through the AV node. The PR interval, when measured, starts at the beginning of the P wave and ends at the beginning of the QRS. Following the PR interval, the ventricles depolarize. This is seen as a tall (or higher) voltage spike, designated as the **QRS** complex. The **Q wave** is by rule the first **negative** deflection after the PR interval, if the first deflection is indeed negative, as sometimes it isn't. In the absence of an initial negative deflection, the Q designation may be dropped. (We often do not drop it, though, and just refer to the electrical event representing ventricular depolarization as the QRS anyway.) The **R wave** is the first positive deflection following the PR interval. The **S wave** is the second negative deflection, if there is a second negative deflection. This can become confusing; however, it should be quite clear later.

Following the QRS, there is a delay until the next wave or deflection occurs. This delay leads into another wave, called the **T wave**. The T wave represents ventricular **repolarization**. The time interval from the beginning of the QRS to the end of the T wave is important and is called the **QT interval**. It is measured from the beginning of the QRS to the end of the T wave. Now, look at an EKG and see whether you can identify these parts.

At the end of the T wave, there might be an additional **low-voltage** deflection. This deflection is called the **U wave**. The U wave, according to experts, represents Purkinje fiber or papillary muscle repolarization, depending on whom you want to believe. The papillary muscles are the small muscles inside the left ventricle that contract to allow the mitral valve to operate properly. The mitral valve is the one-way valve between the left atrium and the left ventricle. It lets blood pass into the left ventricle, but will not allow blood to backtrack through it (see fig. 8).

Figure 8. One cardiac cycle.

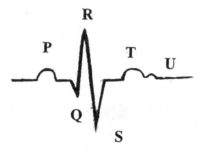

CHAPTER 2: INTERPRETING EKGS

Having mastered the basic principle thus far, the Bonehead is now prepared to start interpreting EKGs. As you will experience later, much information can be obtained from each electrocardiogram—you can't tell what the patient had for breakfast, though. To assist you with organizing your thoughts, we have provided the following list of important observations you should try to note on most of the EKGs you read. It might be helpful to write these down and carry them with you for a while so you won't forget too many of them. It's funny how you can't find something when you don't know what you are looking for.

1. Rate
2. Rhythm
3. Electrical axis
4. P wave configuration
5. PR interval
6. QRS interval
7. QRS complexes
8. ST segments
9. T waves
10. U waves
11. QT duration

The following is a sample form, in part provided by Dr. William P. Nelson and also found in Dr. Marriott's book, *Practical Electrocardiography*. It should be of some help to you. You can even copy and use this form when recording information about the EKGs you are reading. There is no reason why we should have to reinvent the wheel here. The most important part, your overall conclusion after reading the EKG, is listed last. You'll likely be required by your teacher or attending physician to draw some meaningful conclusions from your EKG analysis—if not, why bother reading them?

EKG Evaluation

Make some note of each item

Major EKG parameter	Options	Your conclusion
Atrial and ventricular rate	Normally the same, but they could be different.	
Rhythm	Normal sinus or other?	
P-R interval	Long or short?	
QRS duration	Normal or wide?	
QT interval	Long, short, or normal?	
P wave	Note the shape of the P wave. Abnormalities here could represent left or right atrial enlargement or an ectopic atrial focus.	
QRS axis	Is it pointing in the normal direction? You have to calculate it.	
Abnormal Q waves	In some leads, they're normal, in others, not so normal.	
ST segment	Shifts up or down.	
T wave	Abnormalities—Upright or inappropriately inverted.	
U wave	Present and if so big and obvious?	
Voltages	Small or large? Large could indicate ventricular hypertrophy.	

Now let's learn about each of these parameters so you can understand them.

Rate

Determining the heart rate is relatively simple. You really have to determine two rates, though. Both the atrial rate and the ventricular rate analysis (or calculations) are required. Normally, they are the same, but as you will see, they will differ with some arrhythmias. So how do you go about it? Of course, there is the easiest way, which is to read what the computer thinks the rate is and write that down as the heart rate—not a good idea if you want anyone with half a brain to think you actually know something. Plus, you really can't depend on the computer's accuracy. It's better to be able to do it yourself with alacrity and accuracy. Let's see how we can accomplish that.

With a paper speed of 25 millimeters per second, each horizontal large box is 200 milliseconds. That means that five large boxes is equivalent to one second. Think about that for a second, look at an EKG, and be sure you understand what we just wrote. The standard paper speed of all EKG machines is 25 millimeters per second. One large box equals 5 millimeters; therefore, it takes a duration of one second for five large boxes to scroll across the page. A single QRS spike that happens to occur, every five large boxes will be equivalent to a heart rate of sixty beats per minute, or one beat per second. Remember that five large boxes take up an interval of one second, and there are sixty seconds in a minute. You also might want to know that each large dark box contains five smaller boxes within it. Each smaller box represents an interval of 40 milliseconds. So one large box, composed of five small boxes each representing 40 milliseconds, equates to a total time interval of 40 times 5 to equal 200 milliseconds. Now, think about this. Each large box is the equivalent of 200 milliseconds of time. Notice that it takes five large boxes in a row to make 1,000 milliseconds, which is, of course, one second of time. Do you get this? You have to!

If life were simple every person would have a heart rate of exactly sixty beats per minute, but since life is never simple, we have to have another way to calculate the heart rate of all the EKGs you come across. You guessed it—there is another way, and maybe even more. Just keep reading.

Let's arm you with more brain power to overcome this obstacle. Now try this approach. Locate a QRS complex that falls on a dark vertical line. Then count the number of large boxes until the occurrence of the very next QRS complex. You arrive at the rate by adding the number of large boxes counted between QRS complexes and dividing this number into the number 300. For example, if one large box is counted, the rate is 300 beats per minute—that would be a pretty fast heartbeat. After all, 300 divided by 1 is 300. If two large boxes are counted, the rate would calculate to 150 beats per minute; three, 100; four, 75; five, 60; six, 50; seven, 43; and so on.

If that is too confusing, don't fret—we have yet another way even still. Are you surprised? An alternate method is to count the number of QRS complexes that occur in three seconds. Remember that it takes fifteen large boxes to make a time interval of three seconds, because five boxes equals one second. Now, do the three-second thing and multiply the number of QRSs you see by twenty. For an exact heart rate, divide 1,500 by the number of small boxes between QRS complexes (i.e., 1,500 ÷ 20 small boxes = 75 beats per minute). You get the picture. Now go and practice on an EKG, and then fix yourself a celebratory drink. You are making progress!

The normal heart rate is **60 to 100** beats per minute. Rates less than 60 are referred to as **bradycardia**. Rates greater than 100 are referred to as **tachycardia**. If you don't know these two terms, you are in worse shape than we thought. Never fear; we'll get you up to speed in no time. If we can't, you will always make a fine surgeon! Just remember that "brady" means slow and "tachy" means fast (as opposed to "tacky," like the clothes you wore on your last date).

The Rhythm

Determining what rhythm you think you're looking at can be more difficult. We use the term "think" here, because mistakes are commonly made. As such, this is likely the most difficult topic to teach in the purview of cardiology, and accurate conclusions are often elusive. As usual, we will get you through it easily enough.

The usual rhythm is called a **normal sinus rhythm**. This means that the rate is normal, and the electrical impulse initiates in the usual ("normal") location, which is the SA node. (What follows is just a simple introduction, so don't you get depressed or feel defeated just yet.) If the rate were slow or fast but found its origin within the SA node, where it is normally supposed to, it would be called **sinus bradycardia** or **sinus tachycardia**, respectively. Alternatively, if the electrical impulse originated in the ventricle and was fast, it would be termed **ventricular tachycardia**. We call it "ventricular" because it did not start in the SA node but rather the ventricle (which is abnormal), and we call it tachycardia because it is too dang fast. Again, not normal! As you will see, medicine is full of confusing terms to make it appear more difficult than it really is, but once you understand and familiarize yourself with the jargon, you will be able to figure all this out on your own. If the rhythm originated mostly in the appropriate sinus node but had interspersed occasional ventricular premature beats, it would be called normal sinus rhythm with **ventricular premature beats** (VPBs), sometimes referred to as PVCs. **PVC** stands for **premature ventricular contractions** (they just couldn't wait). The list is long and will be discussed in more detail later; however, some common arrhythmias are illustrated in figures 9–15 to serve as an introduction. Don't worry; we will repeat most of these later. We just want to give you a preview.

Of course, when faced with an almost endless array of combinations and permutations of aberrancy, it is useful to start dividing and classifying things. Lawyers do it, so why can't doctors? Arrhythmias are usually divided into those that originate above the AV node and those that originate below the AV node. Remember that the atria are located above the AV node and the ventricles below it. Those pesky rhythms that originate above the AV node are called **supraventricular arrhythmias**. Those originating below are called **ventricular arrhythmias**. Rhythms that originate within the AV node itself are called **nodal** or **junctional rhythms**. Are you beginning to see how important it is that you know normal anatomy and physiology?

A huge clue as to a patient's rhythm lies in determining whether the rhythm is regular. Regularity means that the P waves and QRS complexes follow a regular and predictable sequence. In other words, they occur rhythmically. You are supposed to see a P wave, then a QRS, then a T wave, and then the sequence repeats itself. It is timely and predictable. Rhythms that are regular include **normal sinus rhythm** and some other rhythms that will be discussed later. Rhythms that are irregular (and there are many that you will come to know) include **atrial fibrillation, chaotic atrial rhythms**, and **atrial flutter** with variable AV conduction. If you are overwhelmed at this point, it's expected. The following examples will help. We'll start with the simple and work our way on down to the more difficult.

Figure 9. Normal sinus rhythm: rate 77 BPM. Note the upright P waves, again indicating the rhythm originates in the SA node. Note the presence of regular as well as narrow predicable QRS complexes.

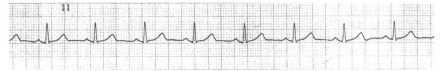

Figure 10. Sinus tachycardia: note same as above, except rate > 100 BPM.

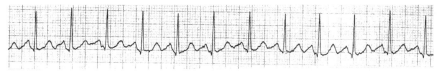

Figure 11. Sinus bradycardia: rate less than 60 BPM; in this case, 44 BPM.

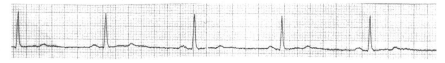

Figure 12. Atrial fibrillation: note the irregular, unpredictable complexes and the absence of discernible "P" waves.

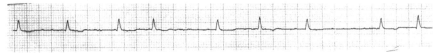

Figure 13. Atrial flutter with variable conduction: note the flutter waves. In this example, adenosine is given to block AV conduction and slow AV conduction to the point where it stops and only atrial flutter waves remain.

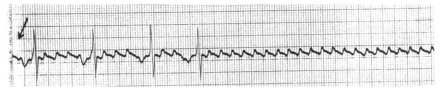

Figure 14. Normal sinus rhythm with PVC: note the W–I–D–E PVC.

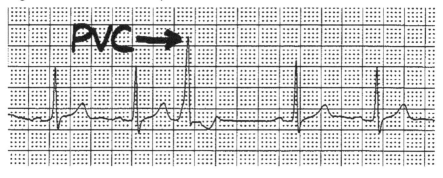

Figure 15. Ventricular tachycardia: note QRS is W–I–D–E throughout and fast. This rhythm originates in the ventricular myocardium and is bad.

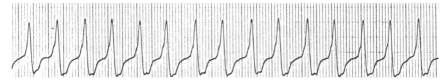

Axis Determination: Using "The Rat"

The electrical axis of the heart should be calculated on each electrocardiogram. The normal QRS axis ranges from negative 30 to positive 90 degrees. Wait! What's this about electrical axis? Sounds a little taxing, we would bet. Why bother you might ask. Because everything that happens on an EKG is a direct result of the intensity, duration, and direction of the electrical activity the heart produces with each beat.

That is how the EKG machine works. It takes all those parameters and variables and measures them and prints it out on the paper for you. A normal heart produces a normal-appearing electrical axis for all of its electrical events. It follows that an abnormal heart would produce abnormal electrical information. Normal or not, the electrical axis is the result on the paper, so you have to understand it.

Axis determination is simple and does not require unnecessary equipment. Incidentally, back in the day, so to speak, pharmaceutical companies would bring lunch to cadres of medical students to tell them about their drugs. They also handed out gadgets with their drug trade names on them to do just about everything but wash your clothes. One of those gadgets was an electrical axis calculator device. You don't need one! To calculate the axis, you should be familiar with how the axis is generated electrically. To do this, you have to understand electrical vectors, so if you thought we had finished talking about vectors, you're having a Bonehead delusion!

Here we go ...

Recall that an EKG electrode records a **positive** deflection if an electrical impulse moves **toward** it. It records a **negative** deflection if an electrical impulse moves **away** from it. It also records an **isoelectric** deflection if the electrical impulse moves at an angle 90 degrees **perpendicular** to it. It follows then, that an upright deflection in lead I indicates that an electrical impulse is moving toward lead I. Would you agree? A negative deflection in AVF indicates that an electrical impulse is going away from AVF. Knowing this, to calculate the electrical axis, you need only to know the location of the electrodes relative to the heart as well as what limb lead has an isoelectric QRS.

Figure 16 uses the **rat model** approach to illustrate the location of the electrodes relative to the heart. What you are about to learn is in no textbook anywhere in publication.

Figure 16. Rat model approach.

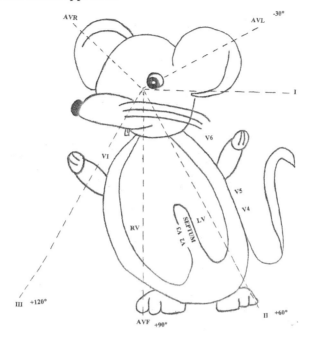

On the rat model, you will notice that the electrode placement is superimposed over the left ventricle, septum, and right ventricle. If you look closely, you will see that they are labeled. Study the picture carefully. Notice that the limb leads I and AVL "look" at the high-lateral wall of the left ventricle. You see them over there just looking and waiting for something to happen. Leads II, III, and AVF look at the inferior wall (bottom) of the heart. That makes sense, because they are located near the rat's feet at the bottom. Note also that V_1 looks primarily at the right ventricle. Leads V_2 and V_3 look at the interventricular septum. You see them sitting right there over the septum. Leads V_4, V_5, and V_6 look at the lateral wall of the left ventricle.

Remember from before that the V leads are looking at the heart in an anterior to posterior direction, or straight through the patient from front to back. Abnormalities in leads V_2 and V_3 will be anteroseptal in location, while abnormalities in V_4, V_5, and V_6 will be anterolateral in location. So when we speak of the V leads, we generally need to add the prefix **antero** when doing so. (Antero means front!)

Abnormalities that occur in the EKG leads II, III, and AVF would indicate pathology at the bottom of the heart. This is because of their location relative to the inferior wall of the heart. Pathology (or changes) seen in leads I and AVL indicate high-lateral wall myocardial disease for the same reason.

You should be getting the sense here that in order to interpret EKGs, it is useful, if not mandatory, to understand where the leads are relative to the various walls of the heart. In speaking of walls of the heart, we are referring to the bottom, left lateral side, anterior side, septal region, and posterior wall. This is where the rat model is most effective. Once you understand this, it will show you where the leads are relative to all the walls, or regions, of the heart.

To get full use of the rat, you need to know how to draw it. Let us teach you how to easily draw it so you don't have to tax your overburdened memory.

If you would rather not learn how to draw it, you can always try to memorize the rather complex figure 17 below. It gives the same information, but you might find it more difficult to learn. Also, it doesn't even locate the other six chest leads (also called V leads) for you. Either way, you have to learn one or the other to be able to read EKGs.

Figure 17. A difficult way to learn the location of the leads around the heart.

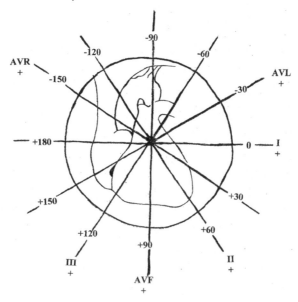

Yes, the rat model is easier to learn than figure 17 that we sort of halfway "borrowed" from a textbook—we just can't recall which one. When drawing the rat, we like to start (and we want you to get a piece of paper and do this step by step with us) by drawing the rat's face. To do this, just draw a circle in the top middle of the paper and put two dots in for makeshift eyes, so you'll be oriented. This will be the rat's face. Actually, it will look more like a mouse, but that's fine. Now draw a crude body on the rat below the face. Tilt the body of the rat to the left side of the paper, or to your right, and make it a little oblong like the one shown in figure 18.

Figure 18. Sequence by which you would draw the rat model.

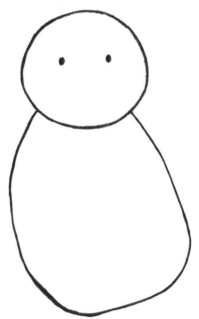

After you have done that, label the parts of the heart by copying what we have diagrammed in figure 19. Note how we labeled the walls of the heart, separating the right ventricle from the left ventricle, and drew in the interventricular septum. Now you have an anatomically correct heart—represented as a rat's body. We know this hasn't taxed you too much. Oh yeah, we also put some mousey-looking ears on the creature for enhancement, and they will be useful to you too.

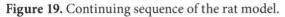

Figure 19. Continuing sequence of the rat model.

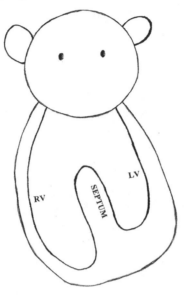

Now we apply the leads to the picture. To do this, we will first draw a whisker to the rat's left side. Start it from just below where you think the rat's nose would be relative to its eyes. Draw it straight to your right, horizontally across the paper. After that, draw two legs. Each leg will go down from the nose. One leg goes to the right, the other to the left, as if the rat were standing with his legs fairly wide apart. Having done that, draw another line straight down from the nose to split the difference between those two legs. This third leg will be perfectly perpendicular to a horizontal line. This will be a three-legged rat. Hang in there, you're almost done. Now, what about those ears on the rat? Draw a line from the nose to bisect the right ear and another from the nose to bisect the left ear. Don't put the ears too high. Now we will label the leads and put some degrees on them so we appear sophisticated. Let's start with that first whisker you drew to the right. Label that lead I. Now go the second lead you drew, which would be the rat's left leg. We will call that lead II. The next lead going clockwise down there is AVF. You know it is AVF because of the "F" in AVF, and because it is close to the rat's **feet.** The next lead, moving clockwise, will be labeled lead III. But where are AVR and AVL? No problem. That's why the rat has ears! The left ear is labeled AVL and the right AVR. Easy, isn't it? Now let's put some degrees on the leads. As you know, circles have 360 degrees in them, and so does the circle you could draw around the rat to intersect all the leads you just drew in. You might think we start counting at zero at the top. If you do, you are wrong. Ha! Just to make it a little confusing, whoever designed this thing decided to let lead I be zero degrees. Going clockwise, lead AVF is positive 90 degrees. That makes lead II positive 60 degrees and lead III positive 120 degrees. If all that is true, then going above lead I toward AVL would make AVL a negative 30 degrees.

Now we have to add the chest, or V leads, to complete the rat. We do not use the V leads to calculate the axis, **only the limb leads**. However, we do want to know what area of the heart the V leads individually see. To locate the V leads, simply put V_1 right over the right ventricular wall. Put V_2 and V_3 over the septum and V_4, V_5, and V_6 over the lateral wall of the left ventricle. Now go back to the rat in figure 19 and see how close you got with the one you drew. You should stop right here and practice this until you can do it without looking. You must be able to get this right. You can't progress until you have an accurate mental picture of this rat, what it represents, and how the EKG leads relate to it.

Figure 20. Completed rat model.

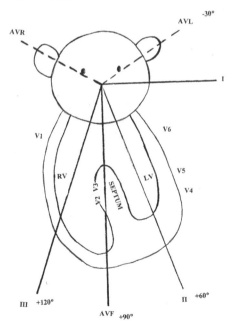

Now let's see how useful this rat can be. The rat model can be instrumental in localizing abnormalities found on the EKG. The abnormalities are then ascribed to their anatomic location on the heart muscle itself. It is also useful and necessary in calculating the electrical axis of the heart.

Now, with that as a background, let's talk about the electrical axis of ventricular depolarization represented on the EKG as a QRS complex (which represents ventricular depolarization). We use no other leads, just leads I, II, III, AVR, AVL, and AVF.

Using the rat model, you can see that if there happens to be an upright deflection in lead AVF and an isoelectric deflection in lead I, then the electrical axis is plus 90 degrees. Now, how did you know that?

Think about the rules we talked about previously. If AVF records an upright deflection, then the electrical vector must be traveling toward AVF, correct? Okay, so that only means that the vector is going to the bottom half of the rat. However, if lead I has an isoelectric deflection, then by prior rules, we know that the electrical vector must be exactly 90 degrees perpendicular to lead I. So what is 90 degrees perpendicular to lead I? Well, it could only go straight up or straight down. We know it doesn't go up. How do we know that? Because if it did, AVF would have to have a negative deflection, and it doesn't. AVF has a positive deflection, so 90 degrees perpendicular to lead I going toward AVF has to be positive 90, or straight toward AVF. You get that?

Now, think of another scenario to further clarify axis calculation. What about an example where there is an upright deflection in lead I? That means the electrical axis is going toward lead I, which is the right half of the rat. Also, in this example, there is an isoelectric deflection in lead AVF. Now where is the axis pointing? The axis, then, is going 90 degrees perpendicular to AVF. It is also going toward the right half of the rat. Recall that the right half of the rat is where lead I is located. The axis, then, would have to be going straight at lead I. Lead I is **zero degrees**.

Another example might reveal the finding of a negative deflection in AVF, an upright deflection in lead I, and an isoelectric deflection in lead II. Working through the process would then reveal an axis that points to minus thirty.

All the previous examples represent a normal axis. The normal electrical axis ranges from **minus 30 to plus 90 degrees**. You could also think of it as going from the rat's left ear to his middle foot. Another way to remember a normal axis is to look at a man directly facing you wearing a necktie. Ask him to pull the tie up and point it to his left ear. Now ask him to drop it straight down to point right over his belly button. The normal electrical axis ranges from his left ear to his belly button. An axis that is in the left upper quadrant of the rat, but above, or more negative than minus 30, is called **left axis deviation**. An axis moved clockwise past straight down and into the lower right quadrant of the rat is called **right axis deviation**. Boneheads can practice calculating axes and become quite proficient using the rat model.

Summary

These are the steps you need to follow to calculate the electrical axis. We suggest you write these down and carry them with you.

1. Check lead I—QRS upright or inverted? If the QRS is upright, then the electrical axis is directed toward the right half of the rat.
2. Check lead AVF—QRS upright or inverted? If the QRS is upright, then the electrical axis is directed toward the lower half of the rat.
3. Locate the isoelectric lead. The final electrical axis is 90 degrees perpendicular to the lead determined by steps 1 and 2 above.

Steps 1 and 2 narrow the electrical axis to a specific quadrant. Step 3 provides the exact axis, as the isoelectric lead is 90 degrees perpendicular to the electrical axis.

Now calculate the electrical axis of the EKG in figure 21:

Figure 21. Illustrative EKG.

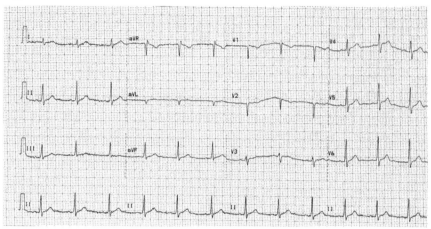

In figure 21, check lead I first and see that the QRS is almost isoelectric. This tells you the axis is 90 degrees perpendicular to lead I. Recall that lead I on the rat is designated 0 degrees. Now look at AVF. The QRS is upright. Therefore, the axis goes toward lead AVF, or the bottom half of the rat, and it is 90 degrees perpendicular to lead I. It is therefore pointing straight at AVF.

Let's try another. Look at the EKG in figure 22 to calculate its axis. First look in lead I. Notice that the QRS is upright. The axis is going to the left half of the rat. Now look in AVF. The QRS is negative. That means the axis is going away from AVF, or to the top half of the rat. Now look for the isoelectric limb lead. Notice that it is lead II in this example. That means the axis is 90 degrees perpendicular to lead II in the left upper quadrant of the rat. It points right at lead AVL. It's not surprising that the QRS in AVL is upright as well. So, the axis in this case is minus 30. Now practice some more on your own, then move on through more of the book.

Figure 22. Another illustrative EKG.

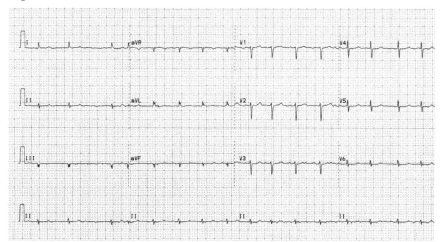

P Waves and Blocks

The P wave represents both right atrial and left atrial depolarization. In the normal P wave, the right atrial component occurs first, followed by the left atrial component. This generally blends into a semibroad P wave with no distinction being made between the right and left atrial components that make up the whole of the P wave. When the left atrium is enlarged, usually because of to LV dysfunction, or possibly hypertension or mitral valve disease, note that the terminal portion of the P wave in lead V_1 becomes **negative** and **broad**. This down-going and broad ending on the P wave in V_1 is called the **P-terminal portion** of the P wave. When this component of the P wave is negative and fills up an entire small box in lead V_1, left atrial enlargement is present. When the P wave becomes wide and notched in the inferior leads, to include II, III, and AVF, then left atrial enlargement is present as well. These are two distinct ways to diagnose left atrial enlargement (see figure 23).

Figure 23. Left atrial enlargement: note arrow. The end of the P wave in lead V₁ is inverted, deep, and wide.

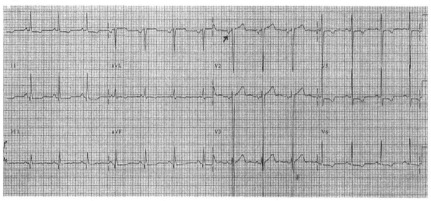

Right atrial enlargement is manifested as peaked, tall-appearing P waves located in the inferior leads, II, III, and AVF. This is because the right atrium sits right over the inferior leads and depolarizes directly toward them. This causes a large upright deflection in these leads. A good rule comes from Dr. Nelson: "If it looks like the P wave would hurt to sit on the P wave in lead II, **there is probably right atrial enlargement present**." Wow, that is a useful "point" we just made. See the example of right atrial enlargement in figure 24.

Figure 24. Right atrial enlargement: note the relatively tall pointed P waves in lead II.

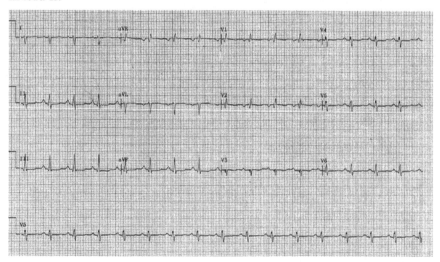

Rules of the electrical axis apply to P waves the same as the QRS. Understand the normal P wave morphology and why it is so by studying figure 25.

Figure 25. Direction of atrial depolarization.

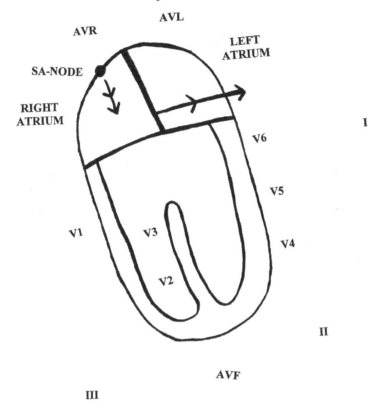

In **left atrial enlargement** (LAE), the terminal part of the P wave (which is the left atrial component of the P wave) in V_1 is negative and wide because the left atrium depolarizes away from lead V_1. Look at figure 25 and prove this to yourself. In a normal heart, what should the P wave look like in AVR? Try to answer without looking at the picture. If the "rat model" is becoming fixed in your brain, you are progressing.

Answer: The P wave must be inverted in AVR because the atria are depolarizing away from AVR. The sinoatrial node, where the atrial impulse begins, is located at the upper portion of the right atrium on the right side. This is where the superior vena cava connects to the right atrium and where a normal "sinus beat" originates. Depolarization of the right atrium must progress inferiorly.

What if you saw an upright P wave in AVR? What do you suppose that would mean? It would mean that you couldn't have a normal sinus rhythm. In normal sinus rhythm, the atria depolarize from the top to the bottom. This must give you a negative P wave in lead AVR.

A **low atrial focus** will also result in an upright P wave in AVR. The term low atrial focus means that a myocardial cell within the atria is electrically impatient—it can't wait to depolarize, so it doesn't. It simply sets off an action potential on its own. Because this abnormal and early depolarization starts at the bottom of the atrium, in this example, it must then travel upward to the top. This sequence is just the reverse of normal sinus rhythm where the depolarization process proceeds from the top to the bottom. Looking at figure 25, you can see how the rat can help you evaluate P waves. The way to use the rat here is to simply divide the rat's face down the middle vertically. The right half of the rat's face now becomes the right atrium and the left half becomes the left atrium. We'll do anything to make it easier for you to learn this stuff!

Atrioventricular Node Blocks

After analyzing the P wave, you should measure the time delay between the beginning of the P wave to the beginning of the QRS. This delay is called the **PR interval**. Just like all intervals, if there is an interval, it's important. Where there is an interval, you can be certain that you're going to have to measure it. Anything that can be measured can be **too long** or **too short**—that's why we measure things, to see whether they're too long or too short.

As an aside, we would like to tell you about a medical student working with a rather intense and insatiable surgeon. The surgeon didn't trust the medical student to do much but cut the sutures as he put them in and tied the knots. The surgeon asked the student to cut the suture, and right after the student cut it, the surgeon barked that the student had cut the suture too long. On the next knot, the student cut again, only to be told that he had cut it too short. This process repeated itself the entire procedure. It was never perfect—always too long or too short. Now, most of us would become unhinged at this point, but this confident medical student strolled into the operating room the next morning to assist the surgeon on the first case of the day. Can you guess what the first thing the student said to this egotistical surgeon when told to cut the sutures again? He replied, "How do you want me to cut them today, too short or too long?" No, the surgeon didn't throw him out of the operating room.

The normal PR interval, which again represents the time it takes the electrical impulse to travel from the atria to the ventricles, is **120–200 milliseconds**. Recall yet again that each tiny little box on the EKG paper represents only a time interval of 40 milliseconds and that there are five tiny boxes in each large box. To measure the PR interval, count little boxes on the EKG paper along the horizontal. Normally, the PR interval will take up a space of three to five little boxes. Three little boxes are 120 milliseconds and five boxes are 200 milliseconds. When the PR interval is longer than 200 milliseconds, or five little horizontal boxes, a **first-degree AV block** is present. Therefore, an EKG that reveals a P wave followed by a QRS that is late in appearing is the definition of first-degree AV block. Now you understand the simplest of AV blocks—but there are more.

Occasionally, the electrical impulse might have more difficulty getting through the AV node. In this case, a P wave might occur with an occasional dropping of a QRS complex. When this happens, this is called **second-degree AV block**. So understand that in the normal heart rhythm, every time a P wave occurs a QRS complex should and must follow. If it doesn't, then there is an electrical block in the AV node that did not let the P wave through.

There are two types of second-degree AV block—**Mobitz I**, also called **Wenckebach block**, and **Mobitz II**. In a Mobitz I second-degree AV block, there is **gradual prolongation of the PR interval** prior to a dropping of a QRS complex. The next P wave, after the dropped beat, will generate a QRS complex with a shorter PR interval. As the P waves continue, the PR interval will progressively lengthen until another QRS is eventually dropped. This is the hallmark of Wenckebach (or Mobitz I) second-degree AV block.

Mobitz II second-degree AV block is more serious than Mobitz I. In Mobitz II second-degree AV block, there is sudden dropping of a QRS complex after the occurrence of a P wave. This failure of AV conduction of the atrial impulse happens unpredictably and **without gradual prolongation of the PR interval**. See the examples in figures 26–30.

Figure 26. First-degree AV block: note long PR interval. Measure from the beginning of the P wave to the beginning of the QRS complex. In this case it is approximately seven little boxes, or 280 milliseconds.

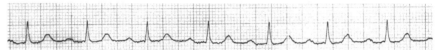

Wenckebach block, also called Mobitz I, occurs when there is a gradual prolongation of the PR interval prior to the dropping of a QRS. After the dropped QRS, the PR interval shortens back to its original length, and the process repeats itself. We realize that this is redundant. Mobitz II block occurs when there's no gradual prolongation of the PR interval and a QRS complex is dropped after a P wave suddenly and without warning. It is important to make the distinction between these two clinical entities, because they have much different implications for the patient's care plan. Just so you know right now, patients who have type I block do not need a pacemaker, while patients who have type II block do.

High-grade AV block requires multiple P waves to cause a QRS complex. Or, said another way, there are at least two P waves seen before a QRS is generated.

Complete AV block, or **third-degree AV block**, occurs when no P waves conduct through the AV node to reach the ventricles. In such a condition, the atrial activity and ventricular activity are seen to be completely independent of each other. The escape rhythm, if there is one, is usually slow and can be narrow or wide. More on that later.

Figure 27. Mobitz I (Wenckebach) second-degree AV block: note gradual prolongation of the PR interval until the QRS is dropped. Then the PR interval shortens back up and starts getting longer again. Think of it as short, longer, longer, then block and back to short.

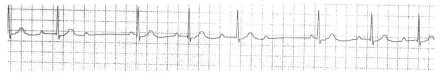

Figure 28. Mobitz II second-degree AV block: coexisting with LBBB in this example. Notice the sudden dropping of a QRS without any PR interval prolongation or warning. This is a potentially dangerous arrhythmia.

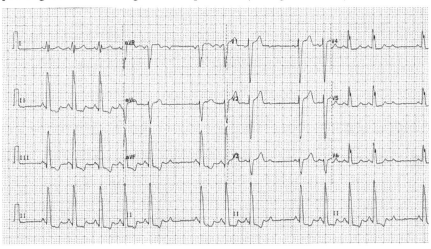

Figure 29. High-grade AV block example: note that more than one P wave is necessary to generate a QRS complex.

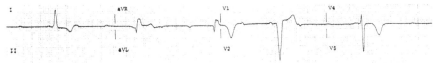

Figure 30. Complete heart block with ventricular escape beats. Note that no P waves conduct through the AV node and that the QRS complexes that do occur are wide.

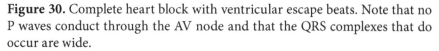

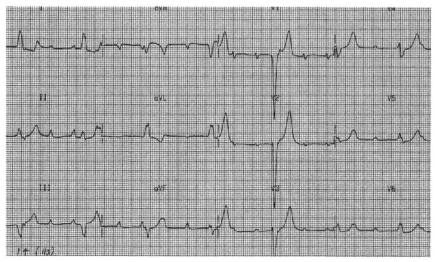

QRS Duration

Normally, the QRS complex is narrow. So, just exactly what do we mean by narrow? By narrow, we mean less than 120 milliseconds. We've already explained why a "normal" QRS is narrow, but it bears repeating. It's narrow because of the unique ability of the specialized conduction tissue in the heart to transmit electrical activity quickly. Recall we talked about the heart's anatomy and the presence of the right and left bundle branches. This tissue allows electrical energy to conduct from one area of the heart to the other extremely fast. As mentioned several times now, the normal QRS duration is normally less than 120 milliseconds. Along the horizontal on the EKG paper, each little box represents 40 milliseconds of time. That means that a normal QRS should occupy three or less small horizontal boxes. If the QRS is wider than 120 milliseconds, then you need to ask why. Conduction abnormalities include **left bundle branch block**, **right bundle branch block**, and **AV node blocks**, already discussed.

In LBBB, the electrical impulse originates in the right atrium and moves down to the AV node. It then continues south through the bundle of His before entering the right bundle branch and passes through with no problem; this is where the problem occurs. The electrical wave finds the left bundle refractory. Refractory means that the left bundle is unable to conduct electricity. This results in normal electrical activation of the right ventricle; however, the left ventricle must wait to receive its activation via myocardial cell-to-cell conduction of electricity from the right side—because the left bundle branch isn't working. As already mentioned, this method of electrical propagation is slow and results in markedly delayed left ventricular activation. A wide QRS complex can easily be predicted. It causes the QRS to appear like the example in figure 31.

Figure 31. 12-lead example of left bundle branch block: note that the QRS is wider than normal. Also notice that the QRS is upright in leads I and V_6 and negative in lead V_1.

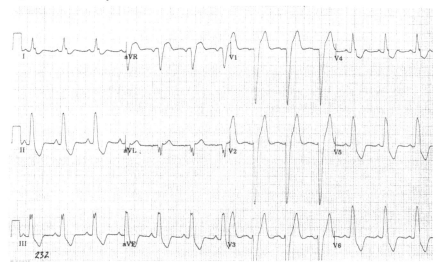

Analogously to left bundle branch block, in **right bundle branch block** (RBBB), the right bundle is broken and can't conduct the electrical impulse. The left bundle, however, continues to function normally. In this situation, the left ventricle fires normally; however, right ventricular depolarization is delayed, resulting in a widened QRS complex. In contrast to a left bundle branch block, right bundle branch block has the morphology noted in figure 32.

Figure 32. 12-lead example of RBBB: note that the terminal part of the QRS is the widest, while the first part is more normal appearing. Also note the up-down-up configuration in lead V$_1$. This is the hallmark of RBBB and is called an RSR' (pronounced r-s-r prime). You might also see the terminal portion of the QRS in lead V$_6$ slurred, and wide.

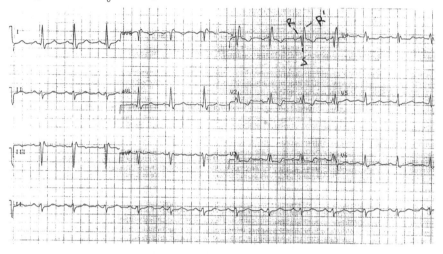

You'll have to distinguish between the two types of bundle branch blocks, so let's help you do that now. Note that in a left bundle branch block, there are wide **upright** deflections in both leads I and V$_6$. In contrast to LBBB, in RBBB, the QRS is wide because of extension of its terminal portion. Also note that the QRS is **negative** in leads I and in V$_6$. In RBBB, there is also a small r wave (the lower-case letter r is used on purpose here because the r wave is small) in lead V$_1$. This is followed by an S wave and then another, taller R wave. This sequence of a small r wave, S wave then large R wave is called an **rSR prime** (rSR), or "**rabbit ear,**" configuration. This is **characteristic of right bundle branch block**. We realize this is redundant, but we want to make sure you understand the difference between the two bundle branch blocks.

Sometimes, QRS complexes are wide because of neither right bundle branch block nor left bundle branch block. When wide beats occur that are not a result of right or left bundle branch blocks, it's likely that the electrical impulse originates at a location within the myocardium itself. If this occurs, you can surmise that there will be slow conduction of the electrical activity and the QRS will be wide. The slow activation causes the QRS to not only be wide, but gives it an appearance similar to a PVC. Figure 33 is a rhythm strip with PVCs.

Figure 33. Rhythm strip sinus with PVC: note how wide the PVCs are relative to the other beats.

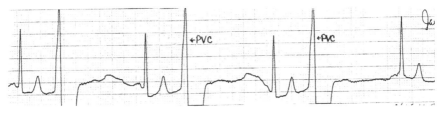

There's one more cause of a widened QRS that you need to be familiar with, and that is aberrant ventricular conduction from the atria to the ventricles through an accessory pathway. Sounds complicated, right? Not really. This is the result of an anatomic anomaly that we'll explore further. This disorder is marked by a **short PR interval** (< 120ms) and a wide QRS. This abnormality is commonly referred to as **preexcitation** and involves an accessory band of muscle tissue, called a **Kent bundle**, which provides an abnormal electrical connection of the atria to the ventricles. This extra band of electrically conducting tissue will allow the atria to activate the ventricles while bypassing the AV node. As the AV node and bundle branches aren't used, the ventricles depolarize aberrantly—resulting in a wide appearing QRS. Aberrant literally means in an abnormal way here.

Understand that normally the only electrical connection between the atria and ventricles is through the AV node. In other words, with the exception of the AV node, the atria and ventricles are electrically insulated from one another. When a band of heart muscle tissue crosses the normally well-insulated atrial-ventricular groove, an electrical impulse has the ability to bypass the AV node and enters the ventricles from the above atria—unimpeded in any way.

Preexcitation is potentially dangerous. Several people have died receiving inappropriate treatment from a physician thinking he was treating ventricular tachycardia when really the patient had a supraventricular arrhythmia aberrantly conducted. Confused? Don't fret; we'll cover this again later. In the meantime, look at figure 34 and pay particular attention to the shorter-than-normal PR interval. Also see there is a slow and slurred upstroke appearance of the QRS, called a **delta wave**. The delta wave appears at the very beginning of the upstroke of the QRS. See figure 34 where the delta wave is marked for your ease of recognition.

Figure 34. 12-lead example of preexcitation, or an accessory pathway. This is also known as Wolff-Parkinson-White syndrome. Note the slurred-appearing upstroke of the QRS in leads I and all the V leads except for the first. See also the very short PR interval.

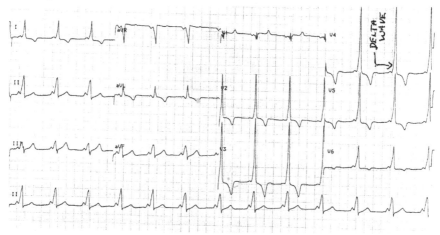

This concludes a cursory introduction to wide QRS complexes. We hope this hasn't been too painful. You don't have to learn it all at one time. Our goal has been to show you how to be able to distinguish between right and left bundle branch blocks. Also, if the QRS is wide, measure the PR interval. If the PR interval is short, then look for the presence of delta waves—you might be the first one to pick up on a case of **Wolff-Parkinson-White syndrome** (WPW). When you think of it this way, it isn't too complicated.

Q Waves

As you go about reading EKGs, you should look carefully at the QRS complex for evidence of prior heart damage—also referred to as a heart attack, or **myocardial infarction** (MI). The presence of pathological Q waves on the EKG usually indicates that a prior myocardial infarction has occurred.

You have to know what Q waves are before you can find them. **Q waves** are **initial negative** deflections of the QRS complex that occur in certain leads. In some leads, Q waves are normal, while in other leads, they are distinctly abnormal. Now we have to teach you how to distinguish pathologic from nonpathologic Q waves.

Normal Q waves, which are nonpathologic, might be found in leads AVR and III, and possibly even V_1. Very **small Q waves** might be seen in the lateral precordial leads V_4, V_5, and V_6. Their presence doesn't indicate that the heart has suffered any damage. In contrast to nonpathologic Q waves, pathologic Q waves are marked by being **wide and deep**. They can occur anywhere large amounts of heart damage have occurred. Remember leads AVR and III are the exception here, where the presence of Q waves is expected and normal. Q waves occurring in the inferior, lateral, or anterolateral leads, indicates prior myocardial damage in those respective locations. The location of the Q waves on the EKG provides incontrovertible evidence where the heart damage has occurred.

Q waves in the **inferior leads (II, III, and AVF)** indicate a previous **inferior wall myocardial infarction**. Q waves in leads **I and AVL** indicate a previous **lateral wall myocardial infarction**. Q waves in leads V_2 and V_3 indicate a previous **anteroseptal myocardial infarction**. Q waves in leads V_4, V_5, and V_6 indicate an old **anterolateral myocardial infarction**. Now would be a good time to look at your "rat model" and visualize where the leads are again relative to the heart walls. If you can conjure up an image in your mind of your "rat model," you won't have to memorize any of this.

You've already learned that not all Q waves are pathologic. What you've yet to learn is that not all pathologic Q waves are necessarily because of a prior myocardial infarction. Oh no, another twist. Life is full of twists. That's right; not all large Q waves mean prior heart damage—we wish it were that simple. For example, you can see pathologic Q waves in patients with **hypertrophic cardiomyopathy** where there has been **no history** of a heart attack. Hypertrophic cardiomyopathy is, if you don't know, a condition where the heart grows to be very thick. It is associated with **sudden death**, arrhythmias, and poor exercise capacity and is generally inherited from a parent. The problem with hypertrophic cardiomyopathy is that most people don't realize they have it until they die. Actually, they never find out, just the bereaved and the pathologist who did the autopsy. We are sure you have heard of young athletes dropping dead for no apparent reason. The occurrence of sudden death in apparently healthy young people is often because of the condition of hypertrophic cardiomyopathy. If you've been paying attention, you have seen that we try to connect facts with physiology. In doing so, we can limit how much you will have to memorize. In that spirit, let us try to help you understand the hows and whys of Q waves.

Fortunately, to help with your understanding of Q waves, we can rely again on our trusty rat model. The development of Q waves is directly related to the change of the electrical axis that results when the heart is damaged—as happens when a heart attack occurs. We told you earlier that you would have to have a clear understanding of the electrical axis, and we meant it. You can see how, if a heart attack has occurred, scar tissue will replace the formerly healthy tissue in the damaged area. This scar tissue is not electrically active. We say it again: **scar tissue is not electrically active**. The area of scarring is unable then to contribute any electrical activity during the heart's contraction. This will ultimately cause an axis shift, which will be apparent on the EKG. So how does this work? Follow along.

In the case of an old inferior wall myocardial infarction, the bottom of the heart has been damaged. The inferior wall, when not damaged, pulls the axis down. In the absence of healthy tissue on the bottom of the heart, the axis will then shift superiorly and laterally. This results in an electrical axis that will be directed **away** from the inferior leads. This axis shift, which results from heart muscle damage, causes and explains the initial negative deflections in the inferior leads (which are Q waves seen in inferior wall myocardial infarctions).

If you're having difficulty, in figure 35 see how on the rat model the dead myocardium on the bottom of the heart fails to pull the axis down; this results in an axis that points **up** and **away** from the inferior leads.

Figure 35. Dead rat example of an inferior wall myocardial infarction.

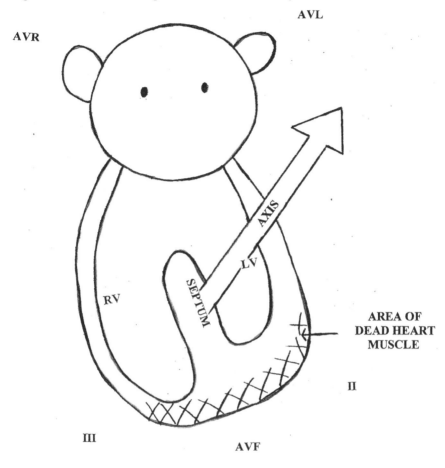

The drawing above illustrates what happens when an inferior wall myocardial infarction occurs. Now let's see what happens with a lateral wall heart attack. You can extrapolate this for yourself and see that if the lateral wall were to be damaged, then the axis would shift almost 180 degrees opposite of where it is in figure 35. Why? Because when the lateral wall is damaged beyond repair, it too will be electrically silent. The rules governing vectors will take effect now and shift the resultant electrical vector away from the lateral wall. It'll have to, because of the presence of unopposed right ventricular and inferior electrical forces. This will cause Q waves to form in the lateral leads, I and AVL, because the electrical new axis will be pointing directly away from these leads. Having trouble? See figure 36.

Figure 36. Dead rat example of a lateral wall myocardial infarction.

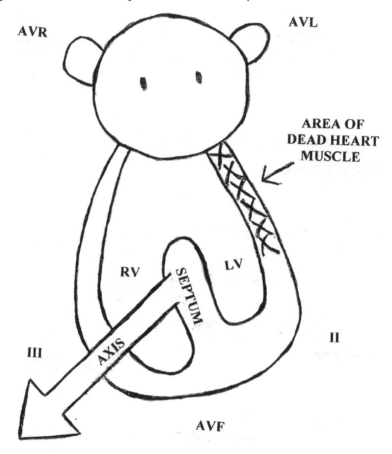

ST Segments

Having discussed Q waves, we'll now transition to ST segments. It's important to pay close attention to the ST segments, because many cardiac abnormalities hide within them. To understand what is abnormal, you first have to be able to recognize what is normal. That makes sense. You'll recall from earlier in the book that the ST segment starts at the end of the QRS and ends at the beginning of the T wave.

Normal ST segments are all aligned horizontally with everything else, including the baselines of the P wave and the T wave. This means that everything is on the same horizontal line. When the ST segments line up with all the aforementioned, they are termed **isoelectric** with the baseline. Shifts, or deviations, of the ST segments from their usual baseline vertically usually indicate that something is wrong. Now, let's look at some specifics regarding ST segment displacement.

In **acute transmural myocardial infarction**, ST segment **elevation** occurs. (By the way, "transmural" just means all the way through the wall of the heart.) You can remember this by thinking that when patients have an acute myocardial infarction, most of them, if not treated quickly, will die. When they die, they usually go to heaven. Most people in the Western world consider heaven to be located up there somewhere. So, simply speaking, when a heart attack occurs, most of the time their ST segments follow them north. If you have no religious inclination, then you can come up with another way to remember it.

We are making a distinction here between acute, which implies occurring right now, and old heart attacks, which are noted by the presence of Q waves on the EKG (we realize the redundancy, but repetition is a great way to learn). As time passes after the heart attack has occurred and the patient is fortunate enough to have survived, the preexisting ST segment elevation returns to its baseline. The exception to this rule is when an aneurysm has formed in the damaged heart wall. This weakened area of heart muscle can, and often does, cause persistent elevation of the ST segments (more on that later).

The take home here is that in acute transmural myocardial infarctions we see **ST segment elevation**.

The term **transmural** means that the damage to the heart muscle is huge—extending all the way from the inside of the heart (called the endocardium) to the outside of the heart (called the epicardium).

Technically, it gets slightly more complicated. Heart attacks that are acute but not extensive, which means that they are limited to just the endocardium of the heart, cause **ST segment depression**. Why, oh why, does this have to seem so complicated? Keep reading. It gets worse!

So large, transmural myocardial infarctions (caused by the acute closure of a coronary artery) result in ST segment elevation, while smaller, nontransmural myocardial infarctions result in ST segment depression. You have to know this distinction. We wish it were as simple as all ST segment elevation means a large heart attack is occurring, but it just isn't so. And it can get even more complicated, but we'll get you through this.

You now know that not all ST segment elevation means acute heart attack. So what else causes the ST segments to elevate?

Sometimes ST segment elevation means heart attack, and sometimes it means something totally different. Let's look at the different causes individually.

One cause is the situation in which there is the occurrence of ST segment elevation in **all the leads** (with the exception of AVR). "**Global ST elevation**" should alert you to the possibility that the patient has **pericarditis**—not an acute coronary thrombosis, which is the fancy way of saying heart attack. So how do you distinguish a good ol' case of pericarditis from a life-threatening heart attack?

In pericarditis, **PR segment depression** occurs along with the ST segment elevation. So if you see ST segment elevation in several noncontiguous leads and become suspicious that pericarditis might be playing a role, look at the PR segments to see if they're sinking below the baseline. If they are, then pericarditis is the likely culprit. This illustrates how important it is to see and talk to the patient too to help you clarify what is wrong and make a diagnosis.

If you are a physician or medical student, it never hurts to take the patient's history and listen to a heart once in a while. The history and physical exam of a patient having a heart attack and one having an episode of pericarditis are dramatically different. Patients with pericarditis typically have a pericardial friction rub that has unique and characteristic sound that a washing machine makes when you hear one working—a to-and-fro sound when you listen to the chest with your stethoscope. Hearing a washing machine sound when you listen to a patient's heart will usually get your attention. Just so you will know, pericarditis is the unfortunate circumstance of having inflammation or an infection of the bag surrounding the heart. This bag is called the pericardium and is prone to all sorts of maladies.

Now back to acute heart attacks. You have to not only know when a patient is having one; you also have to know where it is occurring. As is the case with Q waves and old heart attacks, localizing acute myocardial infarctions follows the same rules—get that rat model back out.

If you were to see ST elevation in leads II, III, and AVF, then you would immediately know that the patient is having an acute inferior wall myocardial infarction. If, on the other hand, you were to see ST segment elevation occurring in leads I and AVL, then you could surmise that the heart attack was affecting the high-lateral wall of the left ventricle.

You will hear much more on this later. Note the example of ST segment elevation occurring in the inferior leads on the EKG in figure 37. This patient is having an acute inferior wall myocardial infarction. Now compare it to another EKG of a patient afflicted with pericarditis printed just below it.

Figure 37. 12-lead example of an acute inferior wall MI with ST segment elevation clearly marked.

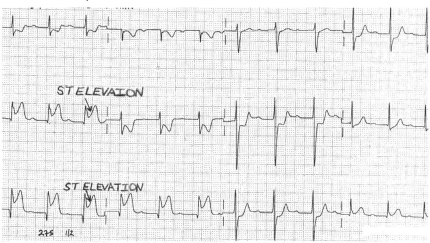

Now look at the EKG example of pericarditis in figure 38. The ST elevation is evident in all the leads, except AVR. Also, if you look closely, you will see PR segment depression, as well.

Figure 38. 12-lead example of acute pericarditis.

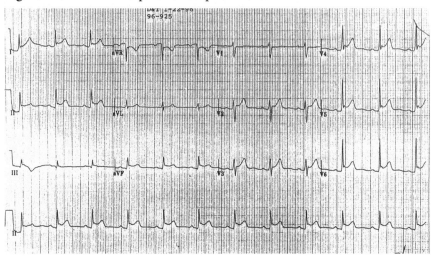

Take plenty of time to study figures 37 and 38. We guarantee that you will see this many times in the future.

For the sake of completeness, we also need to mention that in certain instances, ST segment elevation might not be the result of either pericarditis or myocardial infarction. Oh no, more confusion? Yes, but not much more. Plus, we've already mentioned some of it, so it should be easy.

Sometimes ST segment elevation can occur as a result of an old heart attack that damaged the heart so extensively that it caused the development of a **left ventricular aneurysm**. An aneurysm is an out-pouching of a weakened segment of the muscular wall of the heart that has been previously damaged. It takes a large heart attack to cause the formation of an aneurysm. ST segment elevation associated with a left ventricular aneurysm will persist until the patient dies. This is in stark contrast to ST segment elevation resulting from an acute infarct, which is transient, lasting usually less than twenty-four hours. If you have no old EKG for a comparison, it's easy to confuse an aneurysm with an acute infarct, so always look at an old EKG before you try to interpret the one you have in front of you if at all possible. It just makes your difficult job a little easier. Recall Nelson's Rules we mentioned at the very first part of the book.

Lastly, regarding ST segment elevation, EKGs performed on young

African American males can reveal, curiously enough, ST segment elevation despite their having completely normal hearts. We don't know of anyone who knows how or why this happens sometimes; it just does. Even worse is that the ST segment elevation seen on the EKGs of some young African American men can put on such a convincing show for an acute infarct that even a seasoned cardiologist can be fooled. One defense against being fooled is, again, to make a comparison of the new EKG to the old. No obvious changes of the new compared to the old would indicate a normal variant—nothing to get excited about.

T Waves

You might have noticed that we keep moving the target on you. If you did, you are paying attention. Congratulations! Now we will introduce T waves. You know from prior reading what they are. But just in case you forgot, they represent left and right ventricular **repolarization**. Most of what we have discussed so far has dealt with depolarization. Now we'll look at repolarization.

If you are going to look at the T waves, you might want to know where to find them first. The T wave occurs after the QRS complex. That makes sense. But the T wave doesn't form immediately after the QRS complex. There is a delay between the QRS complex and the T wave. You might recall that this time delay constitutes the ST segment. It's amazing how we have tied these things together, isn't it? We do that for you so that you will have a firm grasp of what we are trying to teach. The T wave is the EKGs electrical recording of the event of ventricular repolarization. All right, so how can we put analysis of the T waves to some useful purpose? Just follow along.

Many physiologic abnormalities reveal themselves in careful observation of the T waves. Not only diseases that affect the heart but also systemic diseases and electrolyte abnormalities can be diagnosed vis-à-vis T wave changes. Let's look at it more closely.

You already know that a QRS complex can be upright or inverted; whether it is one or the other refers to its **polarity**. T waves have polarity just as the QRS does. That means that the T wave can be upright or inverted. You can calculate the T wave axis just as you can calculate the

QRS axis. We won't have you go through all the steps to do that, but it will be helpful to you if you know a few facts about the T wave and its axis.

As a rule, the T wave axis parallels the QRS axis (within 60 degrees). In other words, if the QRS is upright in any given lead, there's a high probability that the T wave should be upright in that lead as well. Conversely, if the QRS is negative, then the T wave should be negative as well (again within 60 degrees).

The T wave polarity follows the QRS polarity as long as the QRS complexes occurred as a result of following the **normal** depolarization process. It is important to realize, however, that when depolarization is abnormal, then repolarization will be abnormal as well. For instance, in the setting of a left bundle branch block, in which the depolarization sequence is abnormal, the T wave will **normally** be directed in a plane **180 degrees opposite** the QRS deflection. In that scenario, an upright QRS should result in a negative T wave. This is opposite the usual case where the QRS and T wave should mirror each other pretty closely. An upright T wave coincident with an upright QRS in the setting of a left bundle branch block is distinctly abnormal. Now, we have said a lot, and we want you to take a moment to digest this. Read it again to make it clear to yourself.

Now that you know what normal T waves should look like, let's see what we can learn from the presence of abnormal T waves. T wave morphology, particularly its polarity, can reveal many things, including the condition of **myocardial ischemia**. When we refer to the myocardium as **ischemic**, we mean that some portion of the heart muscle is not receiving enough blood to meet its physiologic needs. This is almost always associated with a blockage in a coronary artery that feeds the heart muscle freshly oxygenated blood. Saying it another way, inversion of the T waves often results from an ischemic heart. Frequently an ischemic heart is a precursor to a heart attack. So the presence of T wave inversion on an otherwise normal EKG is associated with myocardial ischemia. Simple enough, but it gets a little more complicated.

As is historically the case, there are exceptions to rules, and you must know them. Not all T wave inversion on an EKG is **specific** for myocardial ischemia. Now what do we mean by specific? That simply means that if T wave inversion is present, then ischemia **could** be present. Note we said could be, not has to be.

T wave inversion can also be caused by a long list of other things to include: hypertrophy of the heart, right or left bundle branch block, electrolyte abnormalities, digitalis and numerous other administered drugs, severe hypertension, and central nervous system disorders. That's not a complete list, but it's a good start. So when you see abnormal T wave inversions, think of ischemia as a cause, but be cognizant that there are other illnesses and physical aberrations that can cause the same thing.

Now look at the twelve-lead EKG example in figure 39 that demonstrates T wave inversion across the precordial leads. In the example, see that the QRS complexes in the lateral chest leads are upright, but the T waves are inverted. Look closer and see that T waves are not only inverted, but they are specifically asymmetrically inverted. You have to look carefully, but when you do, you will see that if you folded the inverted T wave exactly down the middle over on itself, the two halves would not be exact mirror images. **Asymmetric T wave inversion** is often present in a patient with **left ventricular hypertrophy (LVH)**. **Symmetric T wave inversion**, on the other hand, is usually more often seen in patients who have an **ischemic heart muscle**. You might well have to make this distinction someday, but we'll work more on that later.

Figure 39. 12-lead example of LVH with asymetric T wave inversion.

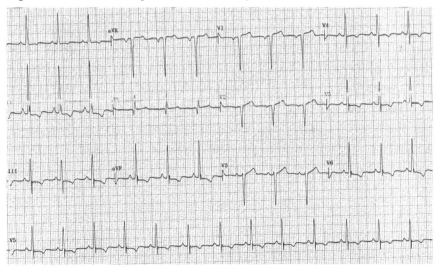

U Wave Analysis

One more wave and we can call it quits with the waves. We bet you're glad to hear that. We have to anticipate the same questions as before, namely, what are U waves and where are they located?

Some cardiac electrophysiologists (doctors who are a lot smarter than us) believe that U waves represent the electrical recording of either papillary muscle or Purkinje system repolarization. We don't really know which of these two really causes U waves, and we don't really care. We don't care because, for our purposes, we don't need to know. How about that! We promised we wouldn't teach you anything you didn't absolutely need to know, and we haven't. We do need to tell you, however, that the U wave occurs just after the T wave—if it occurs at all. What's this "occurs at all" business? Yes, that's right—sometimes U waves are hard to see, ephemeral, or absent altogether. You need to know that they can and sometimes do exist and that you can learn something from them.

To try to make sense of the U waves, we look at their polarity and morphology. In a normal heart, they should be **upright** in the precordial leads. When you think about it, an upright U wave looks more like an "n" wave. If you thought that, you are correct. The one thing about cardiology that you can count on is consistent confusion, and U waves looking like "n" waves should come as no surprise. Out of all this, we want you to take home that the presence of prominent U **waves** is unusual; you should normally have to look really hard to see U waves. When you see them readily, you should think of **hypokalemia** (low serum potassium level). **Inverted U waves** might be present upon your perusal of an EKG. U wave inversion might be a manifestation of **myocardial ischemia**, similar to T wave inversion we have already discussed. Notice the prominent U waves in the EKG shown in figure 40. This patient had a very low potassium level, and the U waves are circled for you to avoid further confusion.

Figure 40. 12-lead example of prominent U waves.

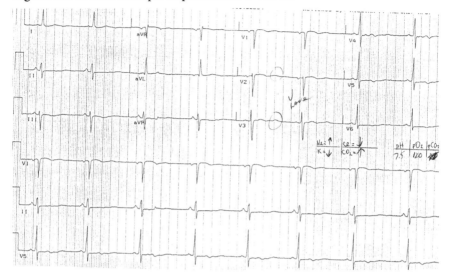

QT Interval

Recall the story of the surgeon and medical student we told you earlier. If you ever become a medical student and find yourself haplessly assisting a seasoned surgeon in the operating room, you'll be asked to cut the sutures after the surgeon ties the knot. In doing so, you will quickly learn that there are only two ways to cut a suture. Those two ways are too long or too short! Whenever you have an interval, it can be too long or too short. So you have to measure it. Of all the intervals mentioned, the QT interval is the most important.

The QT interval is measured as the amount of time that elapses from the onset of the QRS to the end of the T wave. To be clear, the clock starts at the beginning of the QRS and stops at the end of the T wave. This duration of time is normally within the range of 330 to 430 milliseconds long. It can be slightly longer or shorter than the referenced time interval, because it's dependent on the ventricular rate. What we mean by this is that as the **ventricular rate slows down**, the **QT interval prolongs**. As the **ventricular rate increases**, the **QT duration shortens**. So, in effect, the QT duration is inversely proportional to the heart rate. We hope you have that settled in your mind.

It is important to measure the QT interval because a prolonged QT interval might portend a disastrous arrhythmia, called **Torsades de pointes**. This arrhythmia, also known as **polymorphic ventricular tachycardia**, can be life threatening. The various causes of a prolonged QT interval are many and include congenital abnormalities because of chromosomal defects, electrolyte abnormalities, and certain medications. Of the electrolyte abnormalities that prolong the QT interval, hypomagnesemia, hypokalemia, and hypocalcemia are the most prevalent.

In contrast to a prolonged QT interval, shortening of the interval can occur as well. QT shortening doesn't get much press, because it doesn't usually result in life-threatening arrhythmias, but it can reveal the presence of severe hypercalcemia. To illustrate how useful and diverse a tool an EKG can be, let us tell you that we saw a patient at the VA hospital in Columbia, South Carolina, that had a routine EKG done. On the EKG, we noticed a very short QT interval. This alerted us to the possibility of an elevated calcium level, so we checked it. Sure enough, it was 12. That's way too high, and the patient had a bone cancer called multiple myeloma, which raises calcium levels. He would likely have gone a long time not knowing why he felt so bad had we not taken the extra step.

So exactly how should you measure the QT interval? A quick method to assess the QT length is to determine how long the QT interval is relative to the preceding R-R cycle length. If it is longer than half the distance between the two preceding and consecutive R waves, then it is probably too long. Another way to say this is that **the QT interval should always be shorter than half the distance between the two QRS complexes that immediately precede it**. When you measure it this way, you don't have to worry about the heart rate, because you are measuring the proportional length of the QT interval as it compares to the existing heart rate. You don't have to do any real calculations or record any actual numbers. We prefer to do it the easy way, but if you want to be more sophisticated, go ahead. To do this, you would have to measure and record actual QT interval lengths as you see them and then perform calculations based on the patient's heart rate.

Figure 41. Long QT EKG: although in this example you can't really see it, trust us that the QT interval is longer than half the R-R cycle length. This often results in the potentially fatal arrhythmia known as Torsades de pointes.

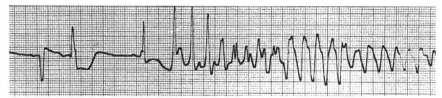

Torsades de pointes means "twisting of the points" in French. As you look at the EKG rhythm strip in figure 41, you can see where the ventricular tachycardia starts. It does so just after the last fairly normal-appearing QRS complex on the leftward side of the strip. The voltage of the ventricular tachycardia beats waxes and wanes, which gives the appearance of a twisting motion in real time. This is an infamous arrhythmia, and you have to be able to know what causes it and diagnose it. We already mentioned electrolyte abnormalities that can cause QT prolongation, but medications can have a similar effect. Some common medications that prolong the QT interval include class I-A antiarrhythmics (which include quinidine, procainamide, and disopyramide), as well as some class III agents (particularly sotalol, amiodarone and others). The commonly used medications Seldane, and erythromycin-type medications, as well as MANY other medications, have the potential to prolong the QT interval and result in Torsades de pointes (Seldane so much so that it has been removed from the market).

Electrolyte Influences on the Electrocardiogram

As you should have already noted, electrolytes can have profound effects on all aspects of the EKG, including the QT interval, the ST segment, QRS complexes, P waves, U waves, and T waves. You will need to be familiar with all of these, so let's start tackling them one by one. We'll start with the common and lethal ones first.

Hypokalemia (low potassium level) causes the U waves to be prominent and the QT interval to lengthen. Recall that a long QT interval can cause death, so that's not good.

Hyperkalemia (elevated potassium level) causes the T waves to change their shape. They become tall and peaked. They sort of have a sharp top to them. Hyperkalemia also causes progressive blunting of the P wave until the P wave becomes absent (if the potassium levels go really high). As hyperkalemia progresses, as it might in kidney failure, the QRS complexes widen and ventricular fibrillation or asystole might result, and you know that's not good either.

Hypomagnesemia (low magnesium level) often causes a prolonged QT interval, so its effects are similar to those of hypokalemia in that respect. In fact, when the QT interval is long and the patient is having rhythm disturbances, we often give them additional magnesium to settle things down. Intravenous magnesium has a soothing effect on an otherwise electrically irritable heart. Incidentally, it is also used by obstetricians to stop preterm labor (we know this isn't a cardiology topic, but we wanted to show you that we are multitalented). We won't mention anything about hypermagnesemia, because you'll rarely see it.

Hypercalcemia (elevated calcium level) causes a shortened QT interval. Short QT intervals don't particularly irritate the heart in any way, but the shortened QT interval as a result of too much serum calcium can readily be diagnosed on an EKG. As we told you before when we were training as cardiology fellows, we once diagnosed a bone disease called multiple myeloma from the appearance of the EKG alone. QT shortening from hypercalcemia is unique in that the QT shortens by reducing the duration of time between the beginning of the QRS to the **onset** of the T wave. This is in contrast to QT shortening due to narrowing of the T wave itself.

Hypocalcemia (low calcium level) causes a prolonged QT interval. As in hypercalcemia, the prolongation of the QT interval is because of lengthening of the QT interval from the beginning of the Q wave to the onset of the T wave. Hypocalcemia doesn't cause the T wave to become wider, as it does in hypokalemia. Do you remember that from a few paragraphs up?

Now, let's look at a few examples (see figs. 42 and 43). Many examples you have already seen, so we won't repeat them.

Figure 42. Example of hyperkalemia: note the peaked appearing T waves.

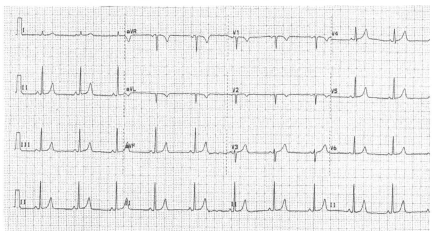

In figure 42, the T waves really aren't that tall; they just look a little too sharp to sit on. This finding implies the condition of hyperkalemia. This brings us to another aside, albeit an important one. Often when we speak of heights of waves, it is not the actual height of the wave that we are literally referring to. We are more concerned with the height of the wave **relative** to the waves around it. For example, if the QRS were abnormally small (meaning having very low voltage), then you would expect the T wave to be proportionally small as well. The finding of T waves that are of "normal" height in the setting of very small QRS complexes might be your only clue to the presence of hyperkalemia.

There are other examples where the relative size of the waves is important and yet has nothing to do with electrolyte abnormalities. These circumstances occur when an EKG is performed on patients who have severe lung disease, obesity, or both. An EKG performed on such a person will likely have small QRS complexes (because of the adipose tissue and trapped air that combine to attenuate the EKG signal). If the QRS complexes are small, then the P waves should be proportionally small as well. If, on this hypothetical EKG, the P waves (in the inferior leads, which look at the right atrium) were of normal size while the QRS complexes were attenuated, then right atrial enlargement would be present. In this case, right atrial enlargement would be present despite the fact that the P waves really didn't actually measure larger than normal. We are just trying to broaden your fund of knowledge and exercise the deductive reasoning portion of your brain. Some people like rules. They need rules and live by them regardless of consequences. They make their lives clearer and simpler. Others, like us, believe that rules are only guidelines, and guidelines are only suggestions.

Figure 43. Example of hypercalcemia: note the short QT interval. The short interval is seen to the onset of the T wave, not in the lengthening of the T wave itself.

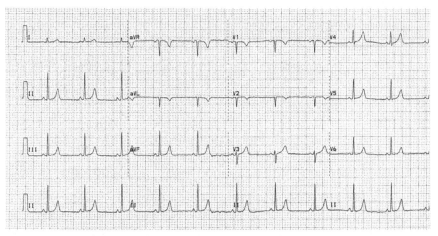

How the Size of the Heart Affects the EKG

You've already learned that the magnitude of a P wave or QRS is proportional to the mass of myocardium depolarizing. If a ventricular chamber of the heart is enlarged, then this enlargement will likely make its presence known by enlarged-appearing QRS complexes on the EKG. Larger-than-normal atria will cause the P waves to appear too big. This is the simple explanation, but we'll need to delve a little further, even as an introduction. We'll address left ventricular enlargement first and then look at what happens when the right ventricle does the same.

There are several methods available to determine if LVH is present, and you can choose whichever method you prefer. This topic can be as simple or complicated as you want to make it. Estes' and Scott's criteria are famous and widely used—so much so that they are published in

Dr. Marriott's book, *Practical Electrocardiography* (see below for Estes' and Scott's criteria). It doesn't really matter which method you use to determine if LVH is present, because they all involve measuring the height of the QRS complexes in some fashion or the other. As Boneheads ourselves, we prefer the easiest of all the ways to evaluate for LVH, so we use Nelson's criteria. (We coined the term "Nelson's criteria," so you won't find it in any other book.)

Nelson's criteria are an easy way to go about ruling in LVH (so much so that we prefer to use it exclusively). They state that LVH is present if the sum of the deepest S wave in V_1 or V_2 (whichever is deeper) and the tallest R wave in V_5 or V_6 (whichever is taller) is equal to or greater than 45 millimeters in height. It also states that this is true if and only if the patient is less than thirty-five years old. In patients older than forty-five years of age, the sum of the deepest S wave and the tallest R wave in the precordial leads need only exceed 35 mm to diagnose LVH. From this, you can extrapolate that a younger patient normally has more voltage on his or her EKG than an older one. You simply can't get any easier than this. You might want to read the above one more time. You are going to have to be able to count and add to do what we suggested.

As stated in his book *Practical Electrocardiography*, Henry J. L. Marriott gives two familiar methods, Estes' criteria and Scott's criteria, to determine whether LVH is present. They are summarized below. These two methods are somewhat involved and require several steps to complete, but they are accurate ways to document the presence of LVH. Each method uses a different scoring system. These scoring systems are excellent and have been used for years, but they might tax your memory a little too much.

Estes' System

Estes' Scoring System for LVH, as the name implies, is a system that involves the accrual of points. The points are given according to specific findings on the EKG. These points are then tallied up at the end. Points are given for the following six findings:

	Finding	Points given
1	R or S in limb lead 20 mm or more	3
	S in V_1, V_2, or V_3 25 mm or more 3	3
	R in V_4, V_5, or V_6 25 mm or more	3
2	Any ST shift (without digitalis)	3
	Typical strain ST-T (without digitalis)	1
3	LAD: –15 degrees or more	2
4	QRS interval: 0.09 seconds or more	1
5	I.D. in V_{5-6}: 0.04 seconds or more	1
6	P-terminal force in V_1 more than 0.04	4
	TOTAL	

If the EKG receives a score of 5 or more, then LVH is present.

A score of 4 reveals likely LVH.

Less than 4, no LVH.

Scott's Criteria

Scott's criteria for determining the presence of LVH is very similar to Estes' criteria, but you don't have to tally. If any of these are present in any of the listed leads, then LVH is present.

Limb leads	Chest leads
R in I and S in III more than 25 mm	S in V_1 or V_2 and R in V_5 or V_6 more than 35 mm
R in AVL more than 7.5 mm	
R in AVF more than 20 mm	R in V_5 or V_6 more than 26 mm
S in AVR more than 14 mm	R and S in any V lead more than 45 mm

By the way, these were borrowed from Marriott's book, previously referenced.

Now let's shift our attention to what happens when the right side of the heart enlarges. **Right ventricular hypertrophy** (RVH) is generally considered a diagnosis of exclusion. Wait a minute. What does that "a diagnosis of exclusion" mean? It means that when we make the diagnosis of RVH, we have to be careful that other unrelated abnormalities don't masquerade as RVH. Needless to say, RVH is a little more difficult to determine with certainty than LVH.

A cursory review of what to expect when RVH is present includes the following: **right axis deviation of the QRS complex** often occurs. It does so because when right ventricular hypertophy is present, the electrical axis must be pulled to the right. This makes sense because the enlarged right ventricle contributes more electrical energy to the QRS vector than usual. Also, as you might surmise, the right ventricle is on the right side of the heart. This larger amount of electrical activity, proportional to the amount of myocardium depolarizing, overwhelms the left ventricular electrical forces and pulls the axis rightward.

You should also know that leads V_1 and V_2 lie almost directly over the right ventricle. Their proximity to the right ventricle gives them a clear view of what's happening on the right side of the heart. In the presence of RVH, there will be **large upright deflections** in these leads. Pull out that "rat" and look at it again.

Secondary causes for right axis deviation, or prominent R waves in leads V_1 and V_2, must be excluded prior to making the diagnosis of RVH. We'll go over all of this later. For now, just review the EKG features of RVH to become familiar with them.

Salient Features of Right Ventricular Hypertrophy (again, according to Dr. Marriot)

1. Reversal of the precordial pattern with tall R over right precordium (V_1, V_2) and deep S over left (V_5, V_6) or S across precordium.
2. QRS interval within normal limits.
3. Late intrinsicoid deflection in V_{1-2}.
4. Right axis deviation.
5. ST segment depression with upward convexity and inverted T waves in right precordial leads (V_{1-2}) and in whichever limb leads show tall R waves.

Conclusion to the Bonehead Basics

Congratulations for making it this far. If you quit now, you would still know much more than most of your colleagues about how to interpret EKGs. By now, you should be convinced that our teaching style is a little different from that to which you might be accustomed. We have to be different—not only to keep your interest, but also to accomplish our goal of helping you become a first-rate EKG interpreter.

We've eschewed memory work and replaced it with a foundation built on having you understand how things work. The simple accomplishment of understanding how things work arms you with the resources necessary for you to complete your EKG education. From here, we can afford to get more sophisticated without causing you any unnecessary confusion. With your new-found knowledge of how an EKG machine works, coupled with your understanding of physics, human anatomy, and physiology, you can make the most of what is to come—and do it with little unreliable memorization work.

We strive to build on your ability to understand and think, as opposed to asking you to memorize an endless sea of different EKG patterns. Pattern recognition will fail you for sure—usually when you need it the most. If you think about it, it is simply impossible to memorize all the abnormal EKG patterns that accompany sick patients, anyway, so that is an untenable strategy. You should be optimistic now that your mission of becoming a competent EKG reader has gotten easier. It is easier because you now have the foundation that those before you never had the opportunity to obtain. You understand how the EKG works.

As we progress, we'll explain in more detail most of what we have just now barely introduced. We'll start our more in-depth look at EKGs with further evaluation and explanation of chamber enlargements (they should be very fresh in your mind). You'll notice that as we continue, we will be using the rat model over and over—so get it out if you don't have it and commit it to memory, so you'll free up your mind to really learn and understand.

CHAPTER 3: HYPERTROPHY (WHEN THINGS GET TOO BIG)

Let's take a minute and review some basic cardiac anatomy and physiology. This information will prove vital as we move along.

You already know that the heart has four pumping chambers, two atria and two ventricles. We know you know this because we have already taught you this. Guess what? We are going to teach it again! Remember that Boneheads like to hear important information more than once, and in different ways.

The atria sit on top of the ventricles. There are four one-way valves present in the normal heart. The **tricuspid valve** sits between the right atrium and right ventricle. The valve between the right ventricle and the pulmonary artery is called the **pulmonic valve**. The valve between the left atrium and the left ventricle is the **mitral valve**. Lastly, the **aortic valve** is between the left ventricle and the aorta. You don't have to memorize all this now, but it will be useful to have a clear understanding of how your heart works. Just know that it has four chambers, each separated by valves and that the upper chambers of the heart are electrically isolated from the lower chambers.

As you learn more about the heart, you quickly realize how form relates to function and vice versa. The heart receives deoxygenated (blue) blood as it returns from the body and reoxygenates it. It then delivers the reoxygenated blood back to the oxygen-hungry organs in the body. The heart is marvelously designed to do its job. Unlike people and other organ systems, the heart can never take a break. It has to work without interruption—or else! Let's look at what happens physiologically in the circulatory system to keep you alive.

Deoxygenated blood from the body returns to the heart through the superior and inferior vena cavae. The superior vena cava drains blood from the head and neck region of the body, while the inferior vena cava drains the lower half of the body. This deoxygenated blood is useless until it replenishes its oxygen content. To accomplish this, it enters into the right upper chamber of the heart, called the right atrium. It pools there until the right atrium contracts, which forces the blood through the tricuspid valve and into the right ventricle below. The right ventricle then pumps it through the pulmonic valve and into the pulmonary arteries as it travels to the lungs. It takes very little pressure for the right ventricle to pump blood through the lungs, because the pulmonary circuit is one of low resistance. It is in the lungs where the blood becomes reoxygenated. The blood then exits the lungs and returns to the heart through the pulmonary veins. These veins carry blood that is now rich in oxygen to the left atrium, where it pools until the left atrium contracts. Left atrial contraction forces the blood down and through the mitral valve and into the very muscular left ventricle below. Because the left ventricle has the job of pumping blood to the entire body, excluding the lungs, it has adapted to its purpose by being thicker and stronger than the right ventricle. It takes tremendous pressure to pump blood from the top of the head to the end of the feet. This is in stark contrast to the right ventricle, which only has to pump the blood through the relatively short and low resistance pulmonary circuit. After filling with blood, the left ventricle contracts, forcing the blood through the one-way aortic valve. When it passes the aortic valve and enters the aorta, it begins its journey to supply the entire body with more oxygen. Ultimately, the blood will reach the tissue level, where the oxygen will again be extracted before the process starts all over again.

We hope that gives you an overview of the circulatory system that is clear and concise. Of course, it's more complicated, but that basic review is all you really need to know.

As mentioned earlier, form and function go hand in hand. Kenyans don't win marathons because they train any harder than Americans. Kenyans win marathons because they are physically different from Americans. Kenyans' leg length to torso length is statistically much longer than that of Americans, giving them much longer strides and allowing them to carry less upper body weight. Offensive linemen on a football team usually don't win the forty-yard dash in time trials. If they wanted to, however, they could increase their chances of being fleet of foot by transforming themselves into sleek, lightning-quick, svelte athletes. Of course, this might require a considerable physical transformation to a much slighter body size. So, when necessary, people can physically change and adapt in form to fit whatever function they aspire to. Football linemen train to become big to push other big people out of the way, and marathon runners try to remain slim so they don't have to carry too much weight over 26.2 miles.

Although the heart, as it comes out of the box, is perfectly designed to do its job, if it encounters unusual resistance, it will adapt—just as athletes adapt. Any of the four chambers of the heart can grow larger. It takes an insult or a hemodynamic load to stimulate the growth of a chamber, but grow it will when required to perform excessive work. We use the term **hypertrophy** to describe the abnormal enlargement of a heart chamber. By looking at the EKG, you can determine if any of the heart's chambers are hypertrophied. We'll now go about teaching you how to do just that. We'll take a look at the two upper chambers of the heart first, including both the right and left atria, and then discuss the lower chambers.

Left atrial enlargement is more common than right atrial enlargement, although they can coexist. Hypertension and malformations or distortions of the normal mitral valve are common causes of LAE. Anything that causes the mitral valve to leak or impedes flow through the valve puts back pressure on the left atrium. This back pressure results in elevated left atrial filling pressure. The left ventricle, as a result of long-standing hypertension, can become stiff and noncompliant. This puts an increased burden on the left atrium as it squeezes to fill the ventricle below. There are many other causes of LAE that we will touch on later, but the most common is hypertension. The hemodynamic consequences of untreated hypertension or a leaky or stenotic mitral valve reflect back to the left atrium in the form of elevated left atrial pressures, which stimulates the left atrium to enlarge.

Chronic lung diseases such as emphysema and asthma are frequent causes of right atrial enlargement. In these diseases, the right ventricle has difficulty pumping blood through the constricted capillaries of the lung vasculature. As the resistance to pulmonary blood flow increases, so does the back pressure on the right ventricle and, ultimately, the right atrium. When the right atrium is exposed to higher-than-normal pressure for a long period, it compensates by enlarging. Some congenital conditions, such as an atrial septal and ventricular septal defect, can cause massive right atrial enlargement.

It shouldn't surprise you that the rat model will help you as you scan the EKG for evidence of right or LAE. We have drawn the rat model in figure 44, but we've altered it a little to help you assess the upper half of the heart for hypertrophy. As you look at the diagram, note the location of the leads relative to the right and left atria.

The rat model will help you most if you are aware of the direction of the electrical vector generated from right and left atrial depolarization—notice that they depolarize in different directions. When you look at the diagram below, which shows all you need to know, you'll see that lead V_1 is almost directly opposite the left atrium. As the diagram shows, the left atrium depolarizes in a direction directly **away** from lead V_1. Note also that leads II, III, and AVF are in perfect locations to see the wave of depolarization generated by the right atrium, as its depolarization wave will approach them **head-on**.

Figure 44. Direction of left and right atrial depolarization relative to the EKG leads.

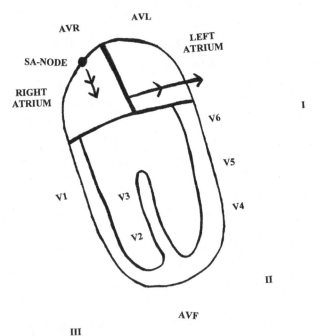

Right Atrial Enlargement

Instead of giving you a menu of EKG findings that occur in the case of right atrial enlargement, we prefer to show you how to discern and predict the abnormalities yourself. It will require you to observe and think, however. Let's start by taking a closer look at the normal right atrium and broaden that discussion to include **right atrial enlargement** (RAE).

Look at figure 44 and see that the right atrium depolarizes from top to bottom. It also sits right over the inferior leads, II, III, and AVF. As the right atrium depolarizes, the mean vector generated travels directly toward leads II, III, and AVF. If you are having trouble conceptualizing this, look at your rat right now. You can then correctly predict, based on the right atrial's direction of depolarization and its location relative to leads II, III, and AVF, that the right atrial component of the P wave should normally be upright in these leads.

Remember that the mass of myocardium depolarizing determines the amplitude (height or voltage) of the wave inscribed on the EKG paper. This is certainly true for the QRS, which represents ventricular depolarization, so it's also true for the P wave, which represents atrial depolarization. Look in leads II, III, and AVF and notice peaked tall P waves that occur in concert with RAE. These P waves would make an uncomfortable seat if you were to sit on them. Dr. Nelson would frequently say to us on rounds, "if it looks like it would hurt to sit on that P-wave, there is right atrial enlargement" See Figure 45.

Figure 45. EKG example of RAE.

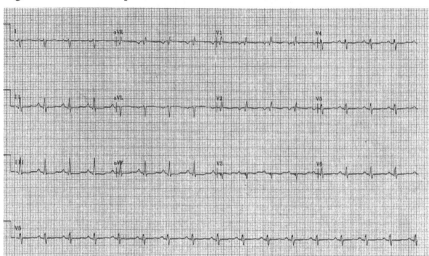

Left Atrial Enlargement

The left atrium depolarizes immediately after right atrial depolarization. Actually, it starts to depolarize while the right atrium depolarizes, but it doesn't finish until after the right atrium has completed the same process. You would think they would depolarize exactly at the same time, but this isn't the case. The left atrium depolarizes just a hair later than the right. Normally, the left atrial component of the P wave is blended in with the right atrial component of the P wave, rendering one solid-looking deflection.

Refer again to figure 44 and see that the left atrium depolarizes toward the patient's left side and down somewhat. Think of left atrial depolarization as heading primarily directly to the patient's left side. Again, this is where the rat model is useful. Referring to figure 44, you will notice that left atrial depolarization, which is traveling to the rat's left side, is oriented directly away from lead V_1. Since lead V_1 observes the electrical impulse generated by the left atrium traveling away from it, it will inscribe a negative deflection on the EKG paper. Remember also that the left atrium depolarizes just ever so slightly after the right atrial activation does. So the left atrial component of the P wave in lead V_1 is the terminal, or second half, of the P wave. It makes sense also that the terminal half of the P wave in lead V_1 will be negative, or downward, because it is depolarizing in a direction *away* from V_1.

You must be able to distinguish the right from the left atrial component of each P wave you see. Referring to the discussion above, the right atrial component of the P wave in lead V_1 will be upright. It's upright because the right atrium is depolarizing directly over lead V_1 and the electrical vector it generates is traveling straight toward it. Recall also that the right atrium depolarizes first. So, when looking at P waves, you notice that the terminal portion of the P wave in lead V_1 is negative (at least one block down and at least one block wide), which is indicative of LAE. To further diagnose LAE, you should look in leads II, III, and AVF for the presence of a **double-humped P wave**. This type of P wave has two crests, or humps. Normally, one solid-appearing P wave is apparent in these leads. However, in **LAE**, the delayed left atrial activation causes the appearance of a delayed second hump of the P wave. The double humps, in order to indicate LAE, have to be separated from each other by at least one small block. See figure 46.

Figure 46. Example of LAE: see the small arrow pointing to the down-going terminal part of the P wave in lead V_1.

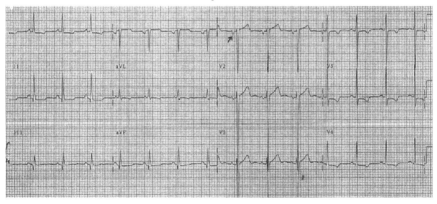

You don't see the double-humped P wave in the inferior leads in this example, but the arrow points to a very clear negative wave at the end of the P wave in lead V_1.

Left Ventricular Enlargement

Now we move inferiorly to the two bottom chambers of the heart. We'll start with the left ventricle and then examine the right.

If you have any curiosity at all, then you are likely interested in what causes **left ventricular enlargement** (LVE). Generally it happens whenever the left ventricle is exposed to greater-than-normal hemodynamic stress. This stress can come from untreated hypertension, obesity, or valvular heart disease, such as mitral and aortic valve stenosis as well as regurgitation of the same structures. Stenosis means that the valve orifice is narrowed or doesn't open properly. This can impede blood flow through the valve, which elevates back pressure. Regurgitation occurs when a valve leaks blood backward. Recall that all four of the heart's valves should function as one-way conduits only. Left ventricular enlargement can be acquired, but it can also be congenital, as is the case with **hypertrophic obstructive cardiomyopathy** (HOCM), **asymmetric septal hypertophy** (ASH), and **idiopathic hypertrophic subaortic stenosis** (IHSS).

As we have mentioned, LVE shows up on the EKG as increased QRS voltage. The big question is how much voltage is too much? You must consider that the patient's body habitus, overall size, lung volumes, and other factors can affect the QRS voltage. You must consider all these variables when determining if a patient's EKG indicates LVE. Also, an unusually thin patient will normally have an EKG that has increased QRS voltage in the absence of LVE.

A series of scoring systems have been devised to score LVE based on probability. These criteria are referred to earlier as Estes' criteria and Scott's criteria. Be advised that we prefer **Nelson's criteria**, hands down, because they are simple. Since we are also Boneheads, we don't expect you to remember too many things at once.

Nelson's criteria state that for a patient less than thirty-five years of age, add the voltage of the S wave in lead V_1 or V_2, whichever is greater, to the tallest R wave in V_5 or V_6. If the total is **greater than 45 mm**, then that patient likely has **LVE**. For a patient more than forty-five years of age, we will allow that total to be only 35 mm. If the total is in excess of 35 mm in the older patient, then that patient likely has

LVE. In addition to this, look in lead AVL alone. **If the voltage of the QRS complex in AVL is greater than 15 mm** (we really love this one because it is one simple sentence), then the patient likely has **left ventricular enlargement**. See figure 47. Also seen are the secondary ST segment and T wave changes often associated with LVE. These secondary changes include inverted T waves and some depression of the ST segments. These changes can occur in any of the leads.

Figure 47. Example of LVH: note the tall QRS complexes and the secondary ST segment and T wave changes.

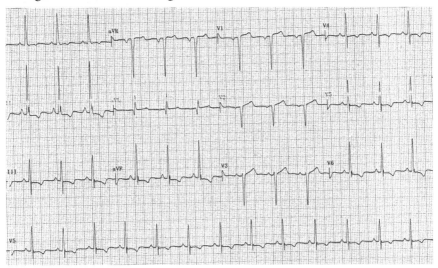

Right Ventricular Enlargement

Fortunately, **right ventricular enlargement** (RVE) is not as common as left ventricular hypertrophy. Lung disease is the most common cause of RVE; the second is occult pulmonary emboli (blood clots that travel from the legs to the lungs). Congenital abnormalities such as an atrial septal defect and pulmonary valve stenosis are also contributors on occasion.

Diagnosing RVE is significantly more difficult than diagnosing LVE. Even experienced electrocardiographers can have difficulty with this one. We won't spend a great deal of time here, because we've already listed for you the salient features of RVE. To help you understand rather than memorize these diagnostic criteria, let us state the following: When you examine the rat model, you will notice that the leads V_1 (and somewhat V_2) are really looking directly at the right ventricle. Go ahead, look at that rat model right now and convince yourself that's true. Right ventricular depolarization is usually overshadowed by left ventricular depolarization. This is because the right ventricle is parchment thin and, as a result, generates very little electricity—compared to the thicker, stronger left ventricle.

When **RVE is present**, the right ventricle depolarizes large myocardial mass. This increased mass generates more electricity during depolarization. This depolarization wave is directed in a vector toward leads V_1 and V_2. As depolarization is traveling toward leads V_1 and V_2, the QRS in these leads will be upright—and prominent! This initial wave of the QRS is seen as a prominent R wave in V_1. There are other factors that might come into play, however, that can and will confuse you—leading to misdiagnosis of RVH. So, you have to pause before giving a patient the diagnosis of RVH when you see a prominent R wave in these leads. Patients might have some other cause of prominent R waves in V_1 and V_2, most commonly a prior **posterior wall myocardial infarction**. Improper placement of the chest leads by the technician is another common mistake that can mimic RVH. There are other circumstances that can lead to the same erroneous conclusion, but if you can remember these two, you're doing fine.

Other abnormalities often accompany RVH, such as **right axis deviation** and incomplete or complete right bundle branch block. These additional findings will help you support a conclusion of RVE on an EKG and give you more assurance that you're correct in your assessment of the same.

A learned doctor named Schamroth (we believe his first name is Leo, but we aren't sure) devised a way of pattern recognition to alert us to the possibility of RVH when certain findings were apparent on an EKG. Our beloved mentor, Dr. Nelson, coined the term **Schamroth sign** when certain results were found on a patient with RVH, including unusually flat—appearing as P, QRS, and T waves in lead I. In fact, all these complexes and waves in Lead I might look very similar to a slightly undulating flat line. These findings tend to occur more frequently when the patient has severe underlying lung disease causing the RVE. The clinical reason for this is that people with lung disease typically have pulmonary hypertension, which causes increased pulmonary vascular resistance. The right side of the heart must overcome this resistance; otherwise, it couldn't pump blood through the lungs. To accomplish this, the right ventricle must hypertophy. See the example of an EKG consistent with RVH in figure 48.

Figure 48. Example of RVH: note right axis deviation and the appearance of an early R wave in leads V_1 and V_2. Notice also the presence of the S wave in the lateral precordial leads.

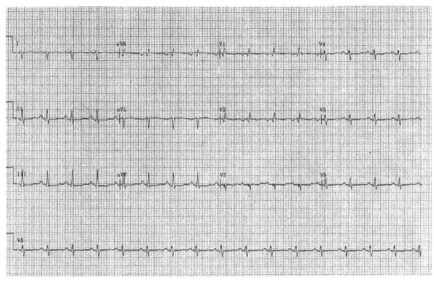

In addition to the early R waves in V_1 and V_2, right axis deviation is also apparent as well as relatively prominent S waves, in V_5 and V_6. If you are observant, you will notice small P waves and T waves in lead I—two findings suggesting Schamroth sign.

CHAPTER 4: RHYTHMS AND ARRHYTHMIAS

As practicing cardiologists for more than twenty years, we still find rhythm determination the most challenging aspect of interpreting EKGs. So, we will now focus on teaching you how to discern what rhythm the patient's EKG reveals. To accomplish this task, you must first understand the normal heart's sequence of electrical activation first. We have covered this already, but we'll review it in case you forgot it or didn't fully grasp it. Either way, now would be a good time for you to review it, before venturing forward. For those of you who are less motivated, we will repeat some critical features below.

To help you recognize arrhythmias, it is important to understand how the normal heart beats. The normal pacemaker for the heart resides in the sinoatrial, or SA, node. This node is physically located at the junction of the superior vena cava and the right atrium. The impulse generated by the SA node makes its exit and activates the right atrium first. This is closely followed by left atrial activation. Although the P wave generally appears as a unified single deflection on the EKG, close inspection might reveal that the two waves of right atrial and left atrial depolarization blend together, appearing as one.

Understand that the P waves in a patient with a normal sinus rhythm will appear upright in leads II, III, and AVF. The reason for this is that these leads view the inferior wall of the heart. Now as the atrial depolarization process starts at the top and travels down toward the bottom, it points directly toward the inferior leads. Conversely, note that in lead AVR (called the oddball lead), the P wave is normally inverted. It is inverted in AVR because the mean vector of atrial depolarization is **away** from AVR. See the normal EKG in figure 49 and prove this to yourself.

Figure 49. Normal EKG: note the upright P waves in leads I, II, III, and AVF and the inverted P waves in AVR.

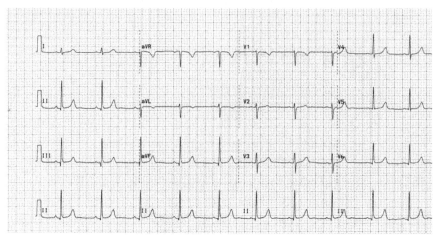

Realize that the polarity of the P waves is not only useful but crucial to determining if the patient's rhythm is normal sinus. If the rhythm originates in the SA node, as it should, the P waves in II, III, and AVF will be upright. Coincidentally with a normal rhythm, AVR will reveal a negative P wave—always. If you find that the P waves aren't oriented this way, then the rhythm isn't sinus—it's something else, a pathological rhythm of some type. Remember this! P wave morphology is the key to determining the patient's rhythm. In order to determine if something is abnormal, you first must know what normal is.

On occasion, reversed polarity of the P waves might represent a problem with the technician who performed the EKG, as opposed to a real problem with the patient. This is seen in the example in figure 50, which is self-explanatory.

Figure 50. Lead misplacement: there is nothing wrong with this patient. The EKG tech reversed the leads, which resulted in inverted P waves in the inferior leads and an upright P wave in AVR.

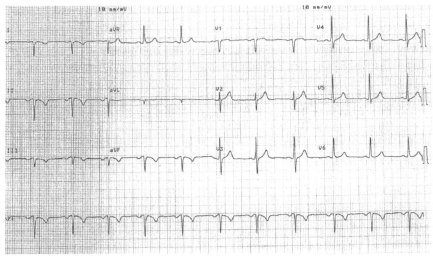

Real-life pathology can result in odd-appearing P waves, as figure 51 demonstrates.

Figure 51. Low ectopic atrial focus: the leads here were placed properly, but the patient has a low atrial rhythm, resulting in P wave polarity reversal. See how the QRS is still negative in AVR, as it should be. In the preceding example, the QRS was upright in AVR.

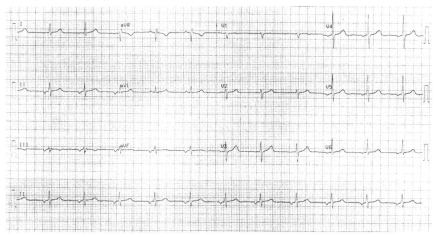

The P waves are sometimes difficult or impossible to see. Rhythms with no apparent P waves certainly are not sinus, as figure 52 below illustrates.

Figure 52. Junctional rhythm: note that there are no discernible P waves prior to any QRS complexes. This rhythm originates within the AV node and is usually less than 60 BPM. There appear to be retrograde P waves within the T waves.

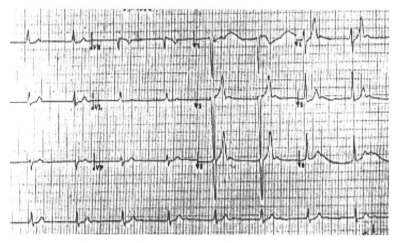

Normal Cardiac Rhythms

Normal cardiac rhythms are just what you expect. Only those rhythms that originate where they should—the SA node—are called **normal sinus rhythms**. Normal sinus rhythms are marked by "normal-appearing P waves." Also, to qualify as a normal rhythm, each P wave must be followed by a QRS every time.

The normal heart rate is defined as being between 60 and 100 beats per minute. **Sinus tachycardia** is a sinus rhythm greater than 100 beats per minute, and **sinus bradycardia** is a sinus rhythm that clicks along at a rate less than 60 beats per minute. Generally, sinus rhythms are quite regular; however, the sinus rhythm occasionally can be somewhat irregular and slightly unpredictable. This circumstance is referred to as **sinus arrhythmia**. This isn't necessarily pathological. The important aspect of sinus arrhythmia to realize is that the P wave morphology will be consistent and normal. This is different from a **wandering atrial focus**, where the P wave morphologies are different. This will be illustrated later.

Arrhythmias

Hold on now! We're going to venture into an enormous morass of problems called arrhythmias. This is a large topic, but not an infinite one. We'll cover most but not all arrhythmias—to do so would require a thousand-page book. And we don't have the time to write one that long.

Arrhythmias that result in superfluous heartbeats are divided into two broad categories: **supraventricular** and **ventricular** dysrhythmias. There might also be combinations of the two. Deletions of heartbeats are also considered arrhythmias. These are the result of electrical blocks in the conduction system somewhere and will be discussed, as well.

To understand arrhythmias better, it is useful to know how arrhythmias come about in the first place. Arrhythmias generally arise from one of two separate pathological mechanisms. First, there might be present an area of the heart that is electrically impatient. That area of the heart muscle just can't wait to depolarize and does so indiscriminately of what the sinoatrial node is doing. While doing this, the impatient focus usurps the sinoatrial node's authority. This phenomenon is called **increased automaticity**. If automaticity occurs in the atria, a premature atrial contraction will result. The early appearing P waves will have a different morphology, or appearance, than the normal P waves of a true sinus rhythm. See the example of sinus rhythm with **premature atrial contractions** (PAC) noted in figure 53. This is an example of a supraventricular arrhythmia because it occurs above the ventricles—in the atria.

Figure 53. Sinus rhythm with premature atrial contractions, or PACs.

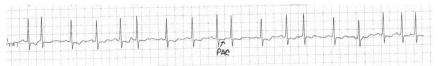

Notice that the QRS following the premature atrial beat is followed by a normal-appearing QRS complex. The early P wave is hard to see, but it's there if you look closely, slightly deforming the T wave.

If the impatient focus originates within the ventricle, a PVC results. See figure 54 below. This is an example of a ventricular arrhythmia. Make note of the fact also that the PVC is wide compared to the QRS following a PAC.

Figure 54. Example of sinus rhythm with PVCs.

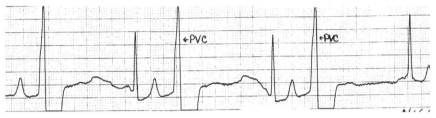

The second mechanism of arrhythmia generation is called a **reentrant phenomenon** or **reentrant loop**. This is quite simple to understand. To form a reentry loop, there must be two separate and distinct pathways through which an electrical impulse can travel. To illustrate this, look at the diagram of the AV node illustrated in figure 55. The atria and ventricles are separated by an electrical—insulating tissue that won't allow an electrical current to pass. The only way an electrical impulse can travel from the atria to the ventricles is through the electrical bridge, called the **AV node**. The AV node is the only electrical connection between the atria and the ventricles in the normal heart.

The AV node in a completely normal individual is a one-lane system where an electrical impulse travels from top to bottom. It looks histologically like a single pathway; however, functionally in the pathological state, two separate pathways exist. A descending electrical impulse can travel through either of the two pathways. These two lanes are distinct and have different properties reflecting variances in **conduction velocity** and **refractory periods**. Conduction velocity refers to how rapidly an electrical impulse travels through the lane. Refractory period relates to how long it takes the lane to recover once an electrical impulse passes through it.

Figure 55. Conduction through the AV node.

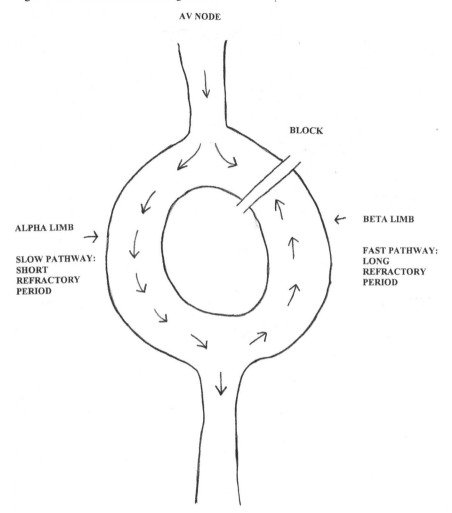

In the examples noted above, notice the AV node is divided into two limbs, designated **alpha** and **beta**. (We don't have to designate them alpha and beta. We could call them anything, really.) The alpha limb properties are such that it is a **slow conductor** of electrical activity but has a very **short recovery period**. The beta limb is a **fast conductor** of electrical activity but has a very **prolonged refractory period**. During the normal sequence of activation, an electrical impulse traveling down through the AV node will split and initially travel through the alpha and beta limbs simultaneously; however, it will exit the beta limb long before it has an opportunity to exit the slower alpha limb. The alpha limb will then not be used. An early electrical impulse timed just so will enter the AV node, and because the impulse is early, it will find the beta limb refractory. By refractory we mean that is unable to carry the electrical impulse. In this circumstance, the electrical impulse will then be forced down the slowly conducting, but quickly recovering, alpha limb. As it conducts, it'll do so slowly. It'll then exit the alpha limb, and by the time it exits, it'll find the beta limb no longer refractory. Finding the beta limb accepting, the impulse can then travel retrograde up the beta limb back up to the atria. The electrical impulse will then reenter the alpha limb because it is a rapidly recovering system, then go inferiorly back down the alpha limb, setting up a reentry loop.

That was a lot of information. You might need to reread what we just wrote to fully understand it. Look at the diagram as you do.

We like to think of this as an electrical impulse chasing its tail, much like a dog chases its tail. Every time the electrical impulse makes the loop, it sends an electrical impulse up toward the atria and an electrical impulse down toward the ventricles. You should probably reread this one more time to cement it in your brain.

If this reentry loop sets up the AV node, it results in **AV nodal reentry tachycardia**, which is discussed further below. If the reentry loop occurs in the atria, within the macro tissue of the atria, then it causes **atrial flutter** to develop. If the reentry loop sets up in the ventricular tissue, it results in **ventricular flutter** or **ventricular tachycardia**. The reentry loop can even set up between the atria and the ventricles themselves, if there's an accessory pathway, as seen in **Wolff-Parkinson-White syndrome**, but we'll discuss this more later.

Now that you understand the pathophysiology of arrhythmia genesis, let's review some common arrhythmias, starting with supraventricular tachycardias.

Supraventricular Tachycardias

As the term suggests, supraventricular tachycardias are tachycardias that originate above the ventricles. So what are the possibilities of areas above the ventricles? This includes the AV node and the atria. We will review them now.

Figure 56. Sinus tachycardia: > 100 BPM.

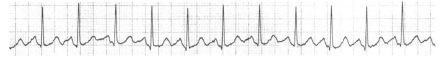

Sinus tachycardia is a sinus rhythm that is going at a rate greater than 100 beats per minute (fig. 56). This is not a true arrhythmia but might be the result of a pathological process in the body somewhere, such as anemia or infection with a fever (fig. 57).

Figure 57. Sinus rhythm with PACs.

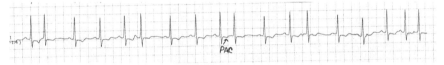

Multifocal Atrial Tachycardia (also called chaotic atrial rhythm)

This arrhythmia originates in the atria and is defined as a heart rate greater than 100 beats per minute and is irregularly irregular. This means that there's no true predictable rhythm to the atrial rhythm. Does that make sense? There is no regularity. Also, the P waves have to have at least **three distinct morphologies**. This implies that there are at least three different areas within the atria firing independently as ectopic atrial foci. This arrhythmia is generally associated with lung disease, hypoxemia, and theophylline toxicity. See figure 58. Note the different P wave morphologies and the rapid and unpredictable rhythm.

Figure 58. 12-lead example of multifocal atrial tachycardia.

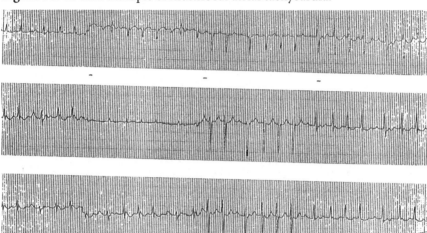

Atrial Flutter

Atrial flutter is, as mentioned, a reentry loop that is set up within the atria themselves. This results in **regular** occurring P waves at about **300 beats per minute**. Not every P wave will make it through the AV node, which is a good thing, because the patient couldn't tolerate a heart rate of 300 beats per minute for very long. Notice the flutter waves in figures 59 and 60. This is a very common arrhythmia.

Figure 59. Atrial flutter with variable conduction: see that there is significant block occurring within the AV node, resulting in many P waves occurring without transmission through the AV node to result in a QRS complex. After the last QRS complex in this example, see the clearly apparent flutter waves that appear as the teeth of a saw.

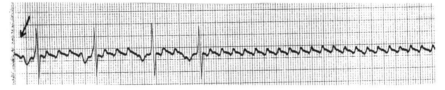

Figure 60. 12-lead atrial flutter: note that in this example the sawtooth pattern is obscured somewhat by the T waves that accompany the QRS complexes. If you look closely, you will see them in the continuous rhythm strip at the bottom of the tracing.

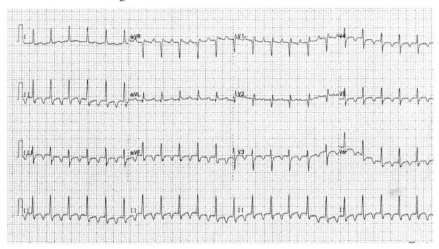

Atrial Fibrillation

Atrial fibrillation is a situation in which the atria are quivering like a bowl full of jelly. Multiple areas are firing and quivering independently at a rate of 300 to 600 times per minute. This usually results in a very coarse undulating baseline with nondiscernible P wave activity. The ventricular response, or QRS complexes, will then be irregularly irregular as well as unpredictable. In addition, the ventricular rate is usually very fast. See the atrial fibrillation example in figures 61 and 62. Notice the irregularly irregular QRSs and the lack of discernible P waves. These are the hallmarks of atrial fibrillation.

Figure 61. Atrial fibrillation: note that there are no discernible P waves. Atrial fibrillation usually has a faster ventricular response than the example below.

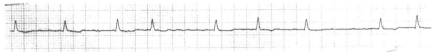

Figure 62. 12-lead example of atrial fibrillation with a rapid ventricular response: note what happens when a drug that slows AV conduction is given.

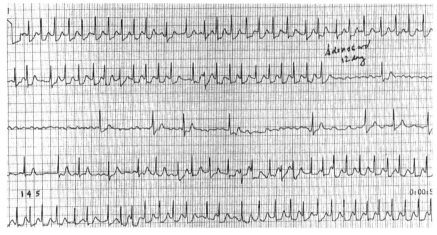

AV Nodal Reentry Tachycardia

This abnormal heart rhythm can be distinguished from atrial flutter, in which the ventricular rate is usually 150 beats per minute, but it can be difficult to do so. In atrial flutter, if the conduction of the atrial impulses through the AV node is two to one, then the ventricular rate is usually 150 beats per minute. In AV nodal reentry tachycardia, the reentry loop is set up within the AV node and results in a regular ventricular rate of about 160 to 200 beats per minute. This is true in most but not all cases of AV nodal reentry tachycardia. As is the case with most supraventricular arrhythmias, the QRS complexes are narrow. If the patient has a bundle branch block, however, the QRS complexes might appear wide, mimicking ventricular tachycardia. It can sometimes be slower and sometimes faster than the speeds mentioned above. You might also be able to see retrograde P waves between the QRS complexes. See figures 63 and 64.

Figure 63. AV nodal reentry tachycardia: this patient's heart rate exceeds 150 BPM, a clue that this is not atrial flutter with 2-to-1 conduction. Careful inspection reveals the presence of retrograde P waves altering the morphology of the ST segments and T waves following each QRS.

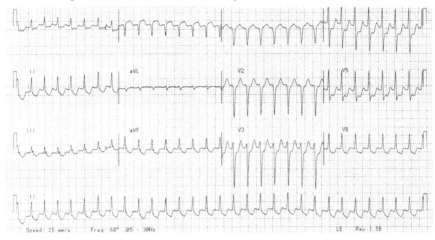

Figure 64. AV nodal reentry tachycardia: note this is easy to confuse with atrial flutter with 2-to-1 conduction, both of which can run at 150 BPM, although AV nodal reentry is usually faster than this.

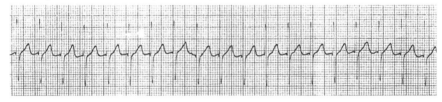

Paroxysmal Atrial Tachycardia (PAT)

This arrhythmia is a result of an ectopic atrial focus firing regularly and rapidly, usurping the sinoatrial node. This arrhythmia is seen quite frequently in digoxin toxic patients. See figure 65 for the example of an ectopic atrial rhythm. PAT will look similar, but with a rate of 100 or greater. Note the inverted P waves in leads II, III, and AVF. This indicates this is not a normal sinus rhythm.

Figure 65. 12-lead example of ectopic atrial rhythm.

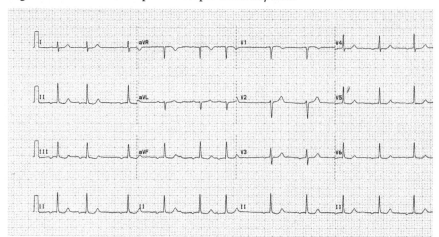

Ventricular Arrhythmias

Premature Ventricular Contractions

Premature ventricular contractions, the most common ventricular arrhythmia you will see, can take many forms. They can be isolated and unifocal (meaning they arise from one location within a ventricle). Unifocal PVCs have a distinct but consistent morphology in any given EKG lead. See the example of a sinus rhythm with isolated PVCs in figure 66. The PVCs are wide and marked and all look the same.

Figure 66. Sinus rhythm with unifocal PVCs.

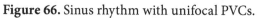

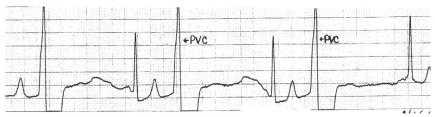

Sinus Rhythm with Bigeminal PVCs
(PVCs that occur every other beat)

See the example in figure 67. If the PVCs came about every third beat, then we would call it trigeminal PVCs.

Figure 67. Sinus rhythm with Bigeminal PVCs.

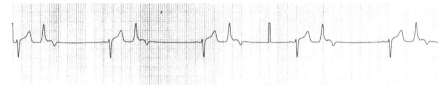

In the above example, the normal beats are narrow and the PVC beats are wide.

Ventricular Tachycardia

This is where PVCs run together in a short or long sequence with no normal beats intervening. They can last for seconds or much longer. Short bursts of consecutive PVCs are called "salvos" of ventricular tachycardia, while long segments of the same are called **sustained ventricular tachycardia**. Note that the ventricular tachycardic beats are wide in the examples in figures 68 and 69 and occur right after the two normal-appearing QRS complexes on the left side of the strip.

Figure 68. Ventricular tachycardia.

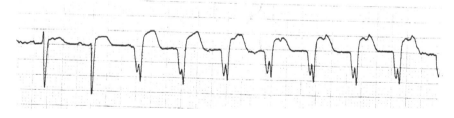

Figure 69. Torsades de pointes: also known as polymorphic ventricular tachycardia, this is a life-threatening rhythm that requires immediate electrical cardioversion. It is a French term meaning "twisting of the points" and is associated with a long QT interval, but not always, as this example shows.

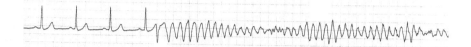

Supraventricular Tachycardias (SVT) Masquerading as Ventricular Tachycardia

These are called the "wide supraventricular tachycardias." They can easily be confused with ventricular tachycardia, so care has to be taken. They're also referred to as supraventricular tachycardia aberrantly conducted. Examples of these are (a) supraventricular tachycardia with a left bundle branch block, (b) atrial fibrillation with a left bundle branch block, (c) supraventricular tachycardia with a right bundle branch block, and (d) supraventricular tachycardias that are conducted through an accessory pathway—as in Wolff-Parkinson-White syndrome. These arrhythmias bring to mind **EKG commandment number IV**: *Thou shall not attempt to interpret an EKG without looking at the patient's prior tracings—if you can get your hands on one.* This commandment sounds simple, but you would be amazed at what lengths some people will go to in order to avoid making a well-informed decision.

See the example of a patient with sinus rhythm and a left bundle branch block in figure 70. The same patient developed supraventricular tachycardia and continued to have the left bundle branch block. The second tracing looks like ventricular tachycardia (fig. 71); however, when referenced with the old tracing, notice that the QRS morphology is identical. This is a clue that this is supraventricular tachycardia with a preexisting left bundle branch block. If you didn't have available the old EKG, you would be inclined to believe that this is ventricular tachycardia, and this would be an erroneous inclination. Boneheads beware! Always attempt to locate an old EKG prior to interpreting the one you are looking at, particularly when an arrhythmia is present.

Figure 70. 12-lead showing normal sinus rhythm with a LBBB.

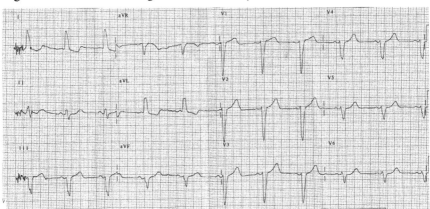

Figure 71. Example of SVT with a LBBB. It looks like V-tach, but it isn't.

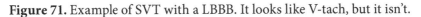

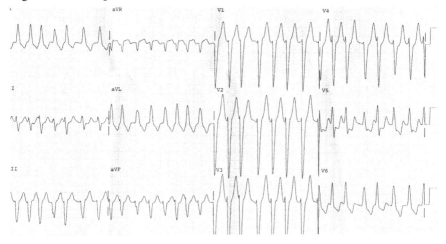

There are many ways to distinguish aberrantly conducted SVT from ventricular tachycardia. The most common way is to search for dissociation of the atrial and ventricular electrical activity (called AV dissociation, where "AV" means atrioventricular). If you can confirm that the ventricles are firing without regard to or in no relation to atrial electrical activity, then ventricular tachycardia is the diagnosis! Often this is difficult or impossible to determine. In such cases, you have to be more sophisticated. This can get complex, so we won't go into any great detail; however, the **wider** the wide QRS is, the more likely it is ventricular tachycardia. Also, 80 percent of the wide complex tachycardias are ventricular tachycardia, while only 20 percent are SVT aberrantly conducted. There are several other methods to help you distinguish the two, but we don't want to confuse you.

Useful Tips and Review of Arrhythmias

It should be apparent that there are numerous rhythm disorders lurking that you'll need to be able to diagnose. If you have a strategy, and you don't panic, you will be right more often than wrong. We suggest you go about the process of determining the rhythm by using the following sequence:

1. Do you see or can you identify any P waves? The absence of P waves guarantees that the rhythm is not sinus. Unfortunately, the presence of P waves doesn't guarantee a rhythm is sinus.
2. Are the P waves associated with ventricular activity? If they are, and the P wave morphology is normal and every P wave is followed by a QRS, then the rhythm is likely sinus. If the P waves are dissociated from the QRS complexes and the QRS complexes are wide, then the rhythm is likely ventricular in origin.
3. Heart rates occurring right at 150 beats per minute strongly suggest atrial flutter with 2-to-1 conduction. Narrow complex tachycardia greater than 150 beats per minute suggests AV nodal reentry tachycardia.
4. Narrow complex tachycardia is always supraventricular in origin.
5. Wide complex tachycardia is ventricular in origin 80 percent of the time, but 20 percent of the time it is supraventricular masquerading as ventricular tachycardia—just to make your job more difficult.

CHAPTER 5: CONDUCTION SYSTEM FAILURE AND BLOCKS

Having read the preceding information, you are now thoroughly prepared to learn more rhythm disturbances called blocks. Electrical blocks can occur throughout the entire conduction system of the heart. These failures in electrical impulse conduction might occur at any time and in any location. Some blocks are physiologic, others pathologic. Once again we draw your attention to the conduction system as it exists in the normal heart. If you forgot it, now is the time to review it. It is important that you have a clear understanding of the normal conduction system prior to attempting to understand electrical blocks.

Recall that a physiological and necessary function of the AV node is to delay the conduction of electricity through it. This will allow the atria enough time to contract and fill the ventricles below prior to ventricular contraction. A full ventricle will be able to expel more blood than a half-empty ventricle.

Physiological block can at times be excessive. When the AV node gets overzealous and blocks the impulse a little too much, the PR interval gets longer than normal. This results in what is termed a **first-degree AV block**. First-degree AV block is a situation in which the PR interval (as measured from the beginning of the P wave to the beginning of the QRS complex) is greater than 200 milliseconds. Two hundred milliseconds is the upper limit of normal for the amount of time it should take an electrical impulse to travel from the atria, through the AV node, and to the ventricles. As stated before, the delay that occurs between atrial and ventricular activation occurs within the AV node itself.

A first-degree AV block might be normal in a well-trained athlete (fig. 72). It can also be caused by diseases and certain medications. Antihypertensive medicines frequently cause some degree of AV block (particularly beta blockers and some calcium channel blockers, as well as clonidine). AV block can also be caused by gradual degeneration of the AV node due to aging. Ischemic heart disease can also contribute to AV block. Other diseases that might contribute to AV block are those that cause deposits to occur in the AV node, such as **amyloid**, **sarcoid**, and **hemachromatosis (an iron storage disease)**.

Figure 72. First-degree AV block: note the long PR interval.

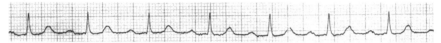

Second-degree AV block is divided into three categories: Mobitz I second-degree AV block, Mobitz II second-degree AV block, and high-grade AV block.

Mobitz I second-degree AV block, also called **Wenckebach block**, is an abnormality that involves progressive prolongation of the PR interval prior to the dropping of a QRS complex (see fig. 73). Remember that in a normal heart, each P wave is followed by a QRS complex every time. In Mobitz I second-degree AV block, subsequent to the dropped beat, the PR interval shortens back to its original length, after which it will progressively lengthen again and eventually result in another dropped QRS. Understand that the hallmark of this block is **gradual prolongation of the PR interval**, culminating in a dropped QRS complex. This phenomenon is physiologic during sleep in some people and can be physiologic in the normal individual. It's no cause for great alarm. See figure 73.

Figure 73. Mobitz I (Wenckebach) second-degree AV block: note the progressive prolongation of the PR interval prior to the dropped QRS complex. After the dropped beat, the PR interval shortens back up.

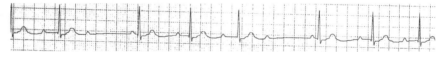

Mobitz II second-degree AV block is somewhat different from Mobitz I second-degree AV block. (Also, you need to know that it has no other name other than Mobitz II second-degree AV block.) Unlike Mobitz I block, the PR interval does not change, and the QRS is dropped suddenly and unexpectedly. So here we have a consistent PR interval and "out-of-the-blue" dropping of a QRS complex. See figure 74.

Figure 74. Mobitz II.

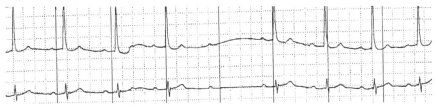

This is a pathological or harmful arrhythmia that will require timely follow-up and attention because a patient with this finding might well progress suddenly to complete heart block. A pacemaker will likely need to be inserted soon into a patient with this problem to prevent syncope (passing out) or even death. Unfortunately, exactly when it will progress to that extent can't be predicted, so anyone with this abnormality should be advised not to drive so as to avoid a calamity.

High-grade AV block is yet another, more ominous, form of second-degree AV block. In this circumstance, it requires multiple P waves to elicit a QRS complex. In other words, it might require two, three, or more successive P waves to "fight" their way through the AV node to spark a QRS complex, which is tantamount to firing the ventricles. In this case, the AV bridge is markedly impaired in its ability to conduct electrical activity; however, it will occasionally and intermittently conduct. This condition is termed high-grade AV block. See figure 75.

Figure 75. High-grade AV block: note that it takes three P waves to cross the AV node and stimulate a QRS complex in this example.

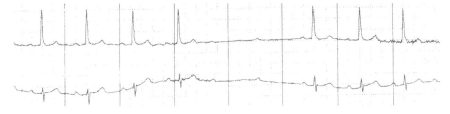

Third-degree AV block, also called **complete heart block**, is a situation in which the AV electrical bridge is completely unable to conduct *any* electrical impulses. This is the most severe of all the different AV blocks. In this setting, the P waves have no ability to conduct through the AV node at all. If a QRS happens to occur in a patient with complete heart block, then it must be the result of an escape mechanism firing at a level below the AV node. See the example of complete heart block in figure 76. The QRS complexes that do occur during complete heart block have no connection to any electrical activity coincident above the AV node.

Figure 76. Complete AV block, or third-degree AV block: note the P waves and the QRS complexes really have no relationship one to the other.

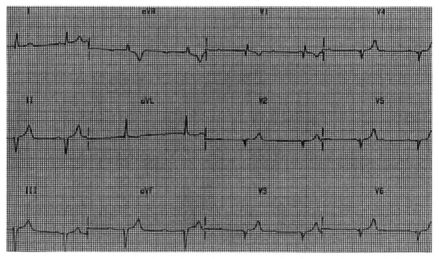

In some cases of complete AV block, the QRS complexes are wide and might have the appearance of a LBBB or linked PVCs. This is determined by where the escape focus is located. If it's high, such as in the bundle of His, the QRS complexes will likely be narrow. If the escape focus is low—for example, originating in the bundles themselves or within the ventricular myocardium itself—the resulting QRS complexes will be wide.

Here is a wonderful opportunity to relate an actual story of something that happened to one of the authors years ago. There was a delightful lady who presented to the office on referral from a primary care doctor for the evaluation of intermittent syncope. She stated that several times over the past year or two she would feel light-headed, then just pass out for a minute or two. She also said that every time she was checked out by a doctor nothing could be found to explain her symptoms. Upon hearing how these severe episodes were affecting her psyche and lifestyle, we decided to put her in the hospital for a couple of days to monitor her heart rhythm and see if we could get to the bottom of the matter. She spent forty-seven and a half hours in the hospital with a monitored rhythm that was as regular and predictable as a pastor showing up at church on Sunday. Just as she was being discharged and we were in her room telling her how sorry we were that we couldn't find anything wrong with her, she said, "Here it comes again!" As we watched, she slowly lost consciousness and stopped talking, breathing, and moving. She also turned a light shade of blue. Then, in fifteen seconds, she woke back up and said she was fine. Quickly, we went to the monitoring station and saw that while she was out, there on the rhythm monitor was evidence that she went over eight seconds without a heartbeat. The monitor strip showed about ten P waves with no QRS complexes. Needless to say, she immediately had a pacemaker implanted. She was the happiest patient to undergo surgery that we had ever seen in our lives. This illustrates how ephemeral and evanescent rhythm disturbances can be at times. Just because a patient's rhythm is normal when you are looking at it, this does not mean that it is normal all the time. Take seriously the complaints your patients make about their body as if you were the patient making complaints to your doctor. All too often, we draw hasty conclusions based on assumptions that are sometimes faulty because of incomplete data. That's just a simple little sage advice we wanted to give that might you help someone in need one day. Ultimately, that is why we become doctors, isn't it?

Bundle Branch Blocks

Having explained the supraventricular and AV node blocks, we will expand our focus and teach you about bundle branch blocks. There are two distinct types of bundle branch blocks, **left bundle branch block** (LBBB) and **right bundle branch block** (RBBB).

If a bundle branch is blocked, whether it is the right or left, then the electrical impulse will travel down the remaining functioning bundle. For the electrical impulse to reach the contralateral side of the heart where the bundle is broken (contralateral means opposite side), it must travel via cell-to-cell conduction of electrical energy. This method of electrical propagation, traveling from cell to cell, is slow and inefficient. It makes perfect sense then that the resulting QRS complex from aberrant, or abnormal conduction, will be wide. Take a moment and think about that.

In order to diagnose either type of bundle branch block, the QRS complex has to be wide. How wide is wide? The answer is **at least 120 milliseconds wide**. Recall that three little blocks on the horizontal of the EKG paper is equivalent to a time interval of 120 milliseconds. The morphology, or shape of the QRS complexes, will determine which bundle is the culprit in causing the block. Now, let's review the distinguishing characteristics of the bundle branch blocks individually.

Right Bundle Branch Block

In the setting of a RBBB, the electrical impulse that originated in the SA node at the superior vena cava right atrial junction travels down the AV node and through the bundle of His. From there, it ultimately reaches both the right and left bundles. Normally, the impulse will travel equally down both of these bundles. In the example of a RBBB, however, the right bundle is physically there—it just is not working. The only option the electrical impulse has is to travel down and through the still-functioning left bundle. As the left bundle is capable of conducting electrical energy, the impulse uses it and travels through it as it should. Upon exiting the left bundle, it first activates the interventricular septum. This activation of the septum occurs in a specific sequence and direction that is important to know.

In RBBB, the septum is activated sequentially from its left side to its right. Because in RBBB the right bundle is nonfunctioning, the left ventricle fires first, and this is closely followed by electrical activation of the right ventricle. This is in contrast to normal heart activation, where right and left ventricular activation are virtually simultaneous.

Reread the above and look at your rat model to be sure that you understand what we have just covered. Because of the unique sequence of electrical activation in RBBB, there is a characteristic RSR configuration noted in the QRS complexes in leads V_1 and V_2, or both. In RBBB, the first upright R wave in V_1, which is smaller than the second upright R wave, is caused by depolarization of the interventricular septum, because this septal activation travels to the patient's right, or your left, toward leads V_1 and V_2. Look at the rat model to lock this image in your mind. Recall that a wave of depolarization traveling toward an electrode causes an upright deflection on the EKG in that lead.

Following septal activation toward the patient's right side—and incidentally again for emphasis, toward V_1 and V_2—the S wave, which follows the initial R wave in RBBB, represents depolarization of the **left** ventricle. This wave of electrical activity necessarily travels away from V_1. The direction of left ventricular depolarization causes the S wave to be negative, or downwardly oriented. And you recall that by definition this negative deflection following an initial upright QRS deflection is called an S wave.

The second upright deflection seen in RBBB is called an R prime (R') wave. It is the result of right ventricular depolarization, which also travels toward V_1 and V_2. This consequential unique morphology of the QRS has been called the **rabbit ear** configuration of leads V_1 or V_2 seen in RBBB (because it looks like a rabbit's ears).

As if that isn't enough, there is more happening to the EKG when a RBBB is present. Also, look in lead V_6, and you will note a slurred and wide-deep negative S wave. Recall that the S wave is the last wave of the QRS complex. This occurs because of late right ventricular activation as a consequence of the RBBB. The delayed right ventricular depolarization travels away from lead V_6, and is seen at the very end of the QRS. After viewing figure 77 below, everything should fall into place for you.

Figure 77. Example of RBBB: note the RSR' configuration of lead V_1 and the delayed and slurred terminal part of the QRS in lead V_6.

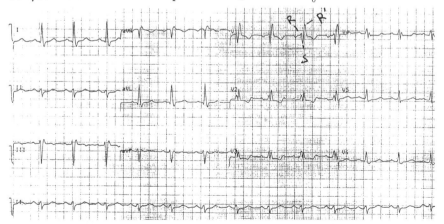

Left Bundle Branch Block

Left bundle branch block is seen as a wide QRS similar to RBBB. In fact, all bundle branch blocks have a wide QRS, which is at least 120 milliseconds long. A nonfunctioning left bundle is distinguished from RBBB in that it doesn't have the "rabbit ear" configuration in leads V_1 or V_2 we just described. Instead, this block's QRS morphology is seen as a wide and upright deflection in leads I and V_6 (recall that RBBB has a slurred, broad S wave in V_6). See figure 78. Recall from the rat model that leads I and V_6 are very close to each other. As a result of their proximity, you can expect the QRS complexes in those leads to appear very similar.

Figure 78. 12-lead of LBBB: note the broad upright QRS in leads I and V_6. Again, all the QRS complexes are wide.

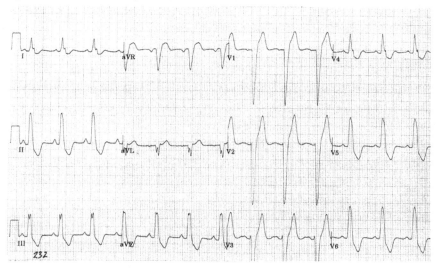

If you are having trouble remembering the difference between RBBB and LBBB, just remember that rabbit ear starts with "R," as does RBBB. Then all you have to remember is which leads to look in, and those are V_1 and V_2—nothing wrong with using a memory aid when available.

Hemiblocks

Hemiblocks can occur only in the left bundle. Why is that? It's because the left bundle is actually composed of **two separate** electrical pathways, also known as fascicles. This is in contradistinction to the right bundle, which consists of only one electrical pathway.

The left bundle is composed of a **left anterior-superior fascicle** and a **left posterior-inferior fascicle**. Both of these fascicles make up what is called the left bundle. Because the left bundle is constructed of two separate pathways, blocks can occur in either or both pathways. If both pathways are blocked, then we have a resultant left bundle branch block. If only the left anterior fascicle is blocked, then we have what is called a **left anterior fascicular block**. If the left posterior fascicle is blocked, then we have a **left posterior fascicular block**. Let's look at these individually.

Left Anterior Fascicular Block (LAFB)

Left anterior fascicular block is noted by a **QRS of normal duration** (that is, the QRS isn't wide), **left axis deviation** (greater than minus thirty degrees), and a **Q wave in AVL**. If the EKG has all three of these findings, then a LAFB is likely present. See figure 79.

Figure 79. EKG example of LAFB: note the normal duration of the QRS the left axis deviation and the small Q wave in AVL.

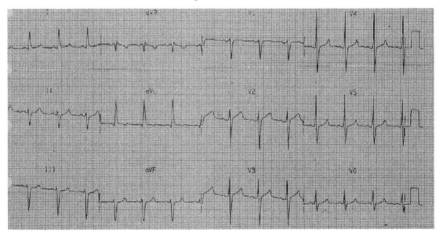

Left Posterior Fascicular Block (LPFB)

Left posterior fascicular block is seen as a QRS of **normal duration**, **right axis deviation**, and the presence of a **Q wave in lead I**. See below for a 12-lead EKG example of a LPFB coexisting with atrial flutter.

Figure 80. Example of LPFB and atrial flutter.

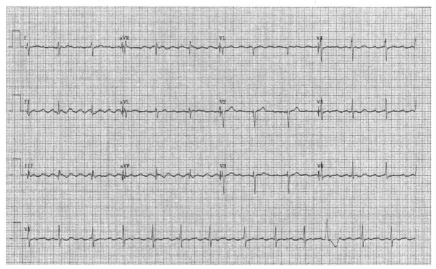

The Q wave in lead I is very small, and the right axis is minimal in this example.

Bifascicular Blocks

Bifascicular blocks are blocks that occur in more than one fascicle, bundle, or location. For example, there could be a RBBB coexisting with a LPFB. Figure 81 is a RBBB coexisting with a LAFB. Notice the RBBB with the RSR prime configuration in lead V_1 and the wide QRS. Also notice the extreme left axis deviation. This is the configuration of an EKG with a RBBB and LAFB.

Figure 81. Example of RBBB and LAFB: note the RBBB along with a left axis deviation and small Q wave in AVL.

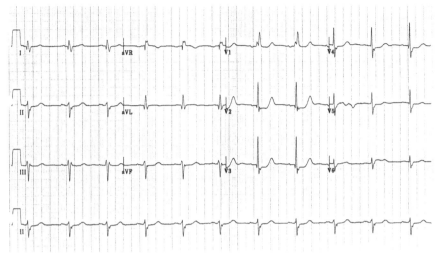

We can also have a RBBB with a left posterior fascicular block (see fig. 82). In this instance, the most dramatic change is the axis shift from leftward to right axis deviation.

Figure 82. Example of RBBB with LPFB.

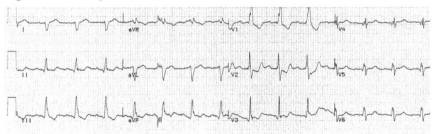

Trifascicular Block

As the name implies, trifascicular block is a block present in three locations. This involves a first-degree AV block in conjunction with either a RBBB and a LAFB, or a first-degree AV block with a right bundle branch block and a left posterior fascicular block. See figure 83 for an example of a trifascicular block.

Figure 83. Example of a trifascicular block: note first-degree AV block, RBBB, and LAFB.

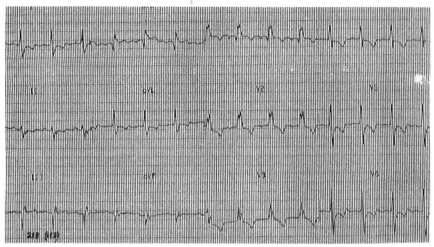

Typically, patients with a trifascicular block have considerable conduction system disease and are well on their way to needing a permanent pacemaker.

CHAPTER 6: MYOCARDIAL INFARCTION AND ISCHEMIA

We wouldn't dare try to teach you anything without first putting what we want you to learn into some context of a real-life situation. In order to accomplish this, we need to educate you a little about myocardial infarction and myocardial ischemia. Let's look at myocardial ischemia first, because it has much milder consequences than myocardial infarction and often forewarns of a more ominous and life-threatening event.

Ischemia is the term used to describe the circumstance of the heart being starved of oxygen-rich blood. Every bodily tissue demands a constant supply of oxygen to function. Continuous uninterrupted flowing blood containing hemoglobin delivers this oxygen efficiently. When an area of the heart receives some but not enough oxygen-rich blood, it becomes ischemic. As the heart becomes ischemic, its ability to function is compromised. This harmful effect can be mild or severe, and the EKG manifestations of the same can be likewise.

Ischemia occurs when a stenosis (blockage) forms in an artery that feeds the heart muscle. If this blockage is greater than 50 percent, it can impede the supply of blood to the heart. If the arterial blockage is severe but not critical, the area of heart muscle supplied by that artery will become ischemic only when it is called upon to work harder than usual, such as when a patient exercises.

When working hard, the skeletal muscles require increased amounts of oxygen. You understand this because when you exercise hard, like running fast, you breathe harder. Working muscles have their oxygen demands met only by asking the heart to pump more liters of blood per minute. This extra pumping action of the heart increases its oxygen demand as well. It also has to have oxygen-rich blood to function at its best.

The heart gets its oxygen supply through a series of arteries sitting on top of it, called the coronary arteries. To illustrate how huge changes in cardiac output can be, consider this. A normal heart with the patient resting pumps about five liters of blood per minute. That's a lot of blood. When that same patient exercises at maximum effort, the heart will pump ten liters per minute—effectively doubling its workload.

A coronary artery with a fixed stenosis can't deliver additional blood on demand to satisfy the extra metabolic demands of the heart when it is put under a load. That is why many patients with heart disease develop symptoms of ischemia (also known as angina) only when they exert themselves heavily but at rest they feel normal.

Myocardial infarction dramatically differs from ischemia, but the physiology is similar—although the EKG findings are not. An infarction occurs when blood flow to an area of the heart is completely interrupted. This usually happens when a preexisting coronary plaque ruptures and the exposed collagen attracts platelets. The platelets then aggregate on top of the plaque and form a blood clot that occludes the artery completely. When this occurs, the affected area of the heart not only becomes ischemic, but it also dies (if blood flow isn't restored quickly). The EKG changes that occur in association with a myocardial infarction are often dramatic and distinct from those that occur in an ischemic situation.

When performed on a patient having chest pain, the EKG can be of its greatest use. It is usual and customary to perform an EKG quickly on any patient having chest pain once they come to an emergency room. Chest pain is the most common physical symptom of a heart attack, but there are many other odd and unusual symptoms that a patient can have that makes the diagnosis of a heart attack less than straightforward. A whole host of strange and elusive symptoms can result from a heart attack. Once we had a patient getting a root canal at the dentist. He told the dentist his jaw was hurting, and sure enough, after the torture of the root canal, he went to the emergency room to see why his jaw still hurt, and it turned out that not only did he get treatment for an abscessed tooth; he also got treated for a huge heart attack. Though you can't rule out a heart attack from a normal-appearing EKG, you can (if the EKG is seriously abnormal) rule one in. To repeat: *A heart attack can't be ruled out by a normal-appearing EKG.* Luckily, though, a full-blown heart attack is usually readily apparent on the EKG—if you know what to look for.

Myocardial ischemia, which again, is a situation in which the heart gets some but not enough blood, can change an EKG from normal to abnormal. Therefore, you have to be able to distinguish between the two. Now we're going to teach you more about the distinct EKG findings in the setting of acute heart attacks and also the changes that commonly occur when a heart becomes ischemic. Just hang in there with us. We will get this all better for you.

Myocardial Ischemia

Consider the clinical scenario of a sixty-year-old male who comes to the office complaining of chest pain that comes on with exertion and is relieved with rest. Assume that this patient's resting EKG is normal. As the patient's physician, you decide that a good diagnostic test would be an exercise treadmill test. The exercise treadmill test is designed to determine if the patient has a significant coronary artery blockage. That obstruction to blood flow becomes apparent with exercise as determined by specific EKG changes.

To determine whether the patient has ischemia, a hemodynamic load has to be placed on the heart. By this, we mean that the heart has to be asked to work much harder than it does in the resting state. One way to accomplish this is with an exercise stress test. The exercise results in increased myocardial oxygen consumption and demand. With a fixed stenosis in a coronary artery, one or more areas of the heart will not get enough oxygenated blood during exercise. These areas that become oxygen depleted during exercise cause changes to occur on a 12-lead EKG. This is exactly why so many exercise stress tests are done each year on those who are "at risk" for heart disease. As an aside, there are many risk factors for heart disease, but the most common are the presence of diabetes, hypertension, high cholesterol, obesity, old age, male sex, and a history of tobacco abuse. There are others, but that's a good start.

Did you know that one third of all patients with heart attacks or severe ischemia have no symptoms? This is particularly true in patients with diabetes. Don't forget that when you see an old man with diabetes complaining of being short of breath with the slightest bit of exertion but no chest pain.

In a patient with a normal heart and no heart disease, the EKG doesn't usually change as the heart rate increases in response to exercise. Fortunately, for those of us who are supposed to be able to diagnose heart disease before a tragedy occurs, there are specific changes that can occur to the ST segments of patients who have significant coronary artery disease and are undergoing a stress test. Let's look at the ST segments more closely and discuss what happens to them when a patient's heart becomes ischemic.

To determine whether a patient has myocardial ischemia, check the ST segments for vertical displacement during the stress test. Assuming the resting EKG is normal, these are evolutionary changes that occur as the workload is incrementally increased. Recall that normally the ST segments are on the "baseline" with the PR segments. Any deviation of the ST segment from the baseline is abnormal.

In an ischemic situation, ST segment displacement can go either up or down. Generally, myocardial ischemia is denoted by **ST segment depression**; however, in extreme cases of ischemia, ST segment elevation can occur. These extreme cases of ischemia (marked by ST segment elevation) are so potentially deadly that they are referred to as **preinfarction** ischemia, because they are often the harbinger of a fatal heart attack.

Now would be a good time to remember that the ST segment begins at the end of the QRS complex and ends at the beginning of the T wave. At the risk of being redundant—this is so important that it bears repeating— realize that the ST segment should normally travel in a horizontal direction and be located exactly on the baseline of the EKG. By horizontal, we mean that the ST segment travels exactly flat across the paper, trending neither up nor down. If you don't know where the baseline is, it is in the same vertical position as the PR segment. During a stress test, if the ST segment becomes depressed, meaning sagging below the baseline, then myocardial ischemia is likely present. If the ST segments trend above the baseline, then ST segment elevation has occurred—and you'll see how worrisome that can be.

The leads in which ST segment changes occur are limited to those leads that "see" the specific area of the heart that has become ischemic. That's good news, because we can use this information to locate specific regions of the heart that are effected by the compromised coronary blood flow. From this information, we can infer not only that the heart is ischemic and where but also what coronary artery has the offending blockage.

In an example where ST segment depression occurs only in the inferior leads, then the ischemia is confined to the inferior wall of the heart. Realize also that the bottom of the heart usually gets its blood supply from the right and occasionally the left circumflex coronary artery. Knowing this, you can infer that either the right coronary artery or the left circumflex artery is effected by a stenosis, or partial blockage. Similarly, if ST segment depression occurs in leads V_5 and V_6, then the ischemia is located in the anterolateral region of the heart. This area of the heart normally gets its blood supply from the left anterior descending coronary artery. We could go on and on with this, but you get the picture. It's just another example of how the rat model will help you anatomically localize the problem.

Figures 84 and 85 are EKGs that were obtained on a patient who, in retrospect, we knew had a high-grade stenosis in a coronary artery. Note the depressed ST segments in the lateral precordial leads and the inferior leads that occurred during the stress test. This was a transient and evolutionary change in the appearance of the EKG that occurred only while the test was being performed. Notice how the ST segment on the exercise EKG takes off from the QRS depressed below the baseline and travels horizontally across the page until the T wave begins.

Figure 84. Example of anterolateral and inferior ischemia on an exercise treadmill test. Note that the resting EKG is normal. 12-lead at rest.

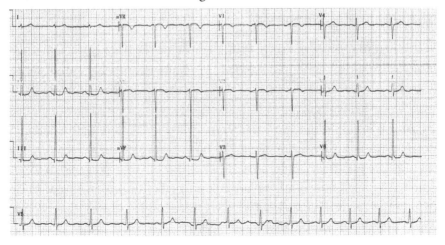

Figure 85. 12-lead with exercise: note the inferior and anterolateral obvious ST segment depression caused by oxygen-starved, hard-working heart muscle.

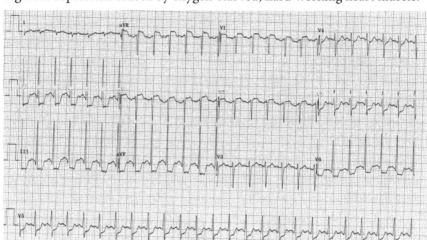

As alluded to earlier, if the heart is subjected to ischemia that is extremely severe, the ST segment might not be depressed at all; instead, in this circumstance, it might become elevated. ST segment elevation during a provocative test, such as an exercise treadmill test, usually indicates extreme myocardial ischemia and requires immediate attention. Note that we don't have an example of this, because everyone we tried this on died and subsequently couldn't sign a release (just kidding).

T Wave Abnormalities in the Context of Myocardial Ischemia

When reading EKGs, it is important to evaluate the T waves for evidence of myocardial ischemia, not just the ST segments. A heart can become ischemic with exercise, but it can also be ischemic at rest if a really tight blockage is present in a coronary artery.

You'll recall from the introductory material that if the QRS is upright, then the T wave will usually be upright as well. This, however, isn't always the case. But it is useful to think of the T wave polarity as paralleling that of the QRS. Reversal of normal QRS and T wave polarity (meaning T wave inversion when the QRS complex is upright and vice versa) might well indicate the presence of resting myocardial ischemia.

This finding of reversed T wave polarity from ischemia is without regard to what the ST segments are doing. So we have two distinct ways to diagnose ischemia: ST segment displacement and T wave changes.

It's not enough to recognize when the T waves are inappropriately inverted; you also have to know **how** they are inverted. They can invert symmetrically or nonsymmetrically (asymmetric). You likely know what symmetric and asymmetric mean, but just in case you don't, think of folding the T wave in perfect half—right down the center. If the two halves are a perfect match, then they are symmetric. If the halves don't match, it is asymmetric.

Symmetric T wave inversion is more ominous than **asymmetric T wave inversion**. Asymmetric T wave inversion is often seen in cases of left ventricular hypertrophy with expected accompanying ST segment changes, which we will discuss later. Symmetric T wave inversion, however, particularly in the absence of LVH, is a fairly frequent and often reliable marker for significant myocardial ischemia, and its presence should pique your interest to investigate things further.

Figures 86–88 are three important EKGs. The first demonstrates the effect of LVH, while the second and third are from the same patient and demonstrate what happens to the T waves when the myocardium becomes ischemic. They are duly noted and explained. Take a good look at them.

Figure 86. 12-lead. LVH with strain: note the inverted T waves and the fact that they appear fairly asymmetric.

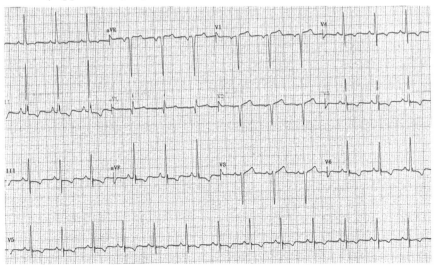

Figure 87. 12-lead with symmetric T wave inversion as seen with myocardial ischemia.

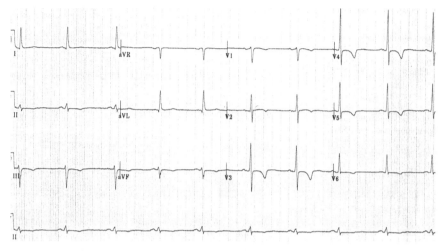

Figure 88. Same patient as above with ischemia resolved after a stent was placed in a coronary artery that had a severe blockage. After the stenting procedure, the T waves have reverted to the upright position.

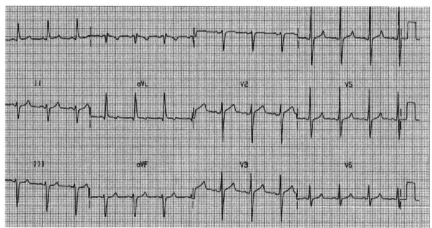

Acute Myocardial Infarction and the EKG

Imagine you're on the golf course and you just missed a two-foot putt for birdie on the eighteenth hole to win the match. Incidentally, you had a lot of money riding on that putt. Just after this, you experience some unusual tightness in the center of your chest. You start sweating profusely and become nauseated. Your playing partners mention that you look a little pale. In a few minutes, you notice that your breath is getting short. What do you think has happened to you? If you guessed that you were having a heart attack, you are right! You now have a 50-50 chance of dying before reaching the nearest hospital. If you take an ambulance there, an EKG will be performed on you in the field and transmitted to the nearest emergency room. Your best hope from here is that the physician in the ER notices the ST segment elevation on the EKG and calls a cardiologist to meet you. Having an EKG there when you arrive will expedite your treatment. Time lost when treating a heart attack equates to heart muscle lost. The more the heart is damaged, the poorer the long-term prognosis. Now is a good time to point out that once a part of the heart muscle is dead, it is dead for life.

The most dramatic manifestation of a large acute myocardial infarction (besides the patient's considerable chest discomfort) is the concomitant ST segment elevation that usually occurs on the EKG. In the setting of acute (meaning occurring right now) myocardial necrosis (which means death of some portion of the heart muscle), the ST segments elevate from their usual baseline. Not only do they transiently elevate, but they elevate in a unique **coved-upwards** appearance. The shape of the ST segments during a heart attack gives them an appearance similar to that of a **tombstone**. That should be easy to remember: coved-upwards, heart attack, and cemetery tombstones all packaged together to tell you that a patient might be having a heart attack. We wish it were this simple, but it isn't.

You should also be aware that ST segment elevation occurs with **most but not all** acute transmural myocardial infarctions (to restate a point made earlier). You would think that all large heart attacks would be apparent on the EKG, but in reality, some are elusive and don't reveal themselves. Oh, why do things have to be so complicated?

When referring to the size of heart attacks, we speak in terms of **transmural** and **nontransmural** to indicate the amount of damage they cause. Transmural is synonymous with big. It is a heart attack that is large enough to result in extensive heart muscle damage. Transmural infarcts are associated with very noticeable EKG changes—especially ST segment elevation. Nontransmural infarcts are small and might not result in any significant ST segment elevation. This reminds us again that you can't rule out a myocardial infarction from the absence of ST segment elevation. A myocardial infarction can, however, be ruled in by the presence of ST segment elevation on the EKG—particularly if you have a normal-appearing old one for a comparison.

One caveat to remember is that pericarditis causes ST segment elevation too, just to throw another monkey wrench into the works. But there are ways to distinguish between the two. In a moment, we'll discuss pericarditis-induced ST elevation and how it compares with myocardial infarction ST segment elevation.

Just as is the case with ischemia, the leads in which the ST segment elevation occurs indicates the area of the heart that is infarcting. For example, if the ST segment elevation were present in the inferior leads— that is, for those of you with short memories, leads II, III, and AVF—the patient is having an acute inferior wall myocardial infarction. If the ST segment elevation occurs in leads V_5 and V_6, it indicates that an acute anterolateral wall myocardial infarction is occurring. If the ST segment elevation is present in leads I and AVL, the patient is having an acute lateral wall myocardial infarction. In figures 89 and 90, we have several examples of patients having acute heart attacks. See whether you can spot the ST segment elevation first, then try to localize where the damage is occurring. You should be starting to really appreciate the utility of the rat that we spent so much time on previously.

Figure 89. Acute inferior infarct: notice the tombstone-shaped ST segment elevation in the inferior leads.

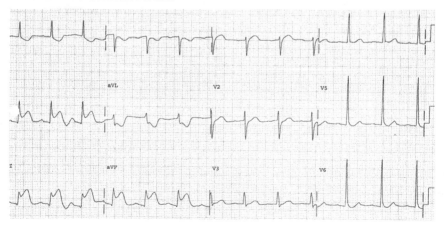

Figure 90. Acute anterolateral infarct: notice the ST segment elevation across the precordial (or chest) leads.

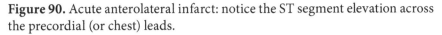

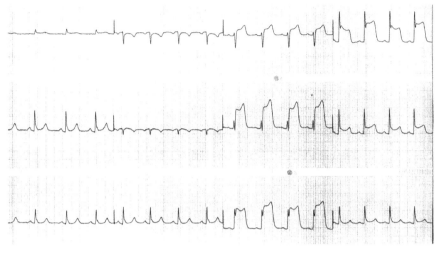

ST segment elevation doesn't always indicate the occurrence of an acute myocardial infarction. If it did, life would be too easy, and your local grocery store clerk could read EKGs. ST segment elevation might also indicate other abnormalities that you have to know, as well. These include both really worrisome and not-so-worrisome conditions. Let's see what those are.

Persistent ST segment elevation—that is, elevation that doesn't go away with time—might be a sign of an **aneurysm** that has formed in the heart. Why would an aneurysm form in the heart, and what is it? An aneurysm occurs when an area of the heart muscle has been damaged from a previous heart attack. This damage would have to have been extensive for an aneurysm to form. During the remodeling process after a heart attack (in which the heart attempts to heal itself), a scar is formed. Since the scar is made mostly of collagen and not muscle tissue, it isn't very strong. Collagen has less tensile strength than muscle as well as an undesirable tendency to stretch over time. It does this when it's exposed to high mechanical pressure—and the heart does produce a lot of pressure as it pumps blood throughout the body. As the collagen scar stretches, it forms an out-pouching. This weakened and stretched-out area of the heart is called an aneurysm. The EKG manifestation of this dangerous situation is persistent ST segment elevation.

So how do you differentiate between ST segment elevation caused by an infarct and ST segment elevation caused by aneurysm formation? ST segment elevation of an acute infarct is transient and will resolve within hours or a couple of days. ST segment elevation caused by the formation of an aneurysm remains for life. This is another situation in which an old EKG for comparison is helpful.

ST segment elevation can also be a normal phenomenon. What's this? We just told you all the horrible things associated with ST segment elevation, and now we say it can be normal? Yes! The specifics of the ST segment elevation, such as its exact shape, can provide you clues as to its cause. If the ST segments are elevated and coved downwards (or scooped out) instead of coved upwards (or convex), then it is possibly a normal variant, although it could still be caused by the malady of pericarditis.

In the case of ST elevation that is a normal variant, it is a result of repolarization changes that are not clearly understood. This situation occurs frequently on EKGs performed on young black men. The ST segments are not coved upward but rather concave in appearance.

Global ST segment elevation which is ST segment elevation affecting all the leads (with the exception of lead AVR) is seen in a condition known as **pericarditis**.

Pericarditis occurs when the bag the heart sits in (called the pericardium) becomes irritated and inflamed. It is painful. The pain tends to worsen when the afflicted patient reclines. Sometimes the pain goes away when the patient sits up. There are physical exam findings in pericarditis that can help you distinguish it from chest pain caused by a heart attack. Patients with pericarditis typically develop a pericardial friction rub that can be heard with a stethoscope. This rub is a distinct, unusual "to-and-fro" sound that is characteristic of pericarditis. It is unforgettable once you hear it because it sounds like the noise that a washing machine makes.

The unique EKG finding in pericarditis (which help the EKG reader know it is pericarditis and not an acute myocardial infarction) is that the PR segment is typically **depressed**. Of course, AVR will be the opposite and have PR segment elevation. This is really the only situation in which you will see PR segment depression, so remember it! Don't be fooled by global ST segment elevation mimicking an all-over myocardial infarction. When you see ST segment elevation in several leads, be sure to look at the PR segments for evidence of depression, as well. See figure 91 for an example of acute pericarditis and compare it to the infarct EKGs that we've already shown you.

Figure 91. Pericarditis: note that the ST segments are elevated in all of the leads except AVR and that careful inspection reveals PR segment depression, as well.

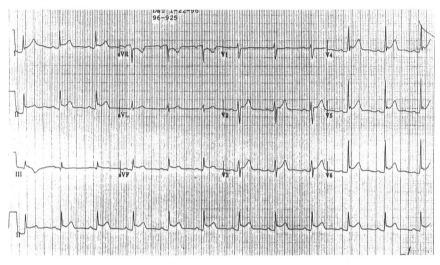

As stated before (but which you may have forgotten, being a Bonehead), you might also notice that the ST segment elevation in pericarditis is concave and not convex. Convex ST segment elevation is more frequent in cases of acute myocardial infarction.

Posterior Wall Myocardial Infarctions: The Great Evader

Every class has to have a clown—a deviant of some type who resists classification and is impossible to predict. Our deviants, when it comes to heart attacks, are posterior wall infarctions. They don't follow the usual rules, so we have to carve out a special class just for them.

We mentioned earlier that not all heart attacks reveal themselves on the EKG. Some are notorious for being elusive. Posterior wall myocardial infarctions can be elusive for sure, but they are worse in that they also violate most of the rules regarding infarcts that we've asked you to learn. Simply put, that means that they reveal themselves on the EKG in unusual ways. You can bet that we are prepared to explain why.

To diagnose posterior myocardial infarctions, you have to understand them. To understand them, you have to forget all that we have already taught you. Not really, but it is opposite of what you would think, and here's why.

By looking at your rat, picture that leads V_1 and V_2 are looking at the right ventricle. The problem is that V_2 is not over the right ventricle on your rat. In your mind, move it from where it is and place it just below V_1. Now you will see that both V_1 and V_2 are looking at the right ventricle. Further inspection, however, will confirm that they're also looking straight through the right ventricle all the way to the posterior wall of the left side of the heart. This is true because the heart doesn't really sit flat in the chest. It is rotated a little to your right or the patient's left, so the left ventricle is closer to the spine, and the right ventricle is closer to the chest wall. It looks flat in the picture, but in three dimensions, it is rotated about 30 degrees.

You have to be able to generate a three-dimensional image of the heart in your head (with the leads superimposed) to fully appreciate this. Remember that the precordial leads (or V leads) look directly through the heart from front to back. And these leads can see and record everything happening in the front of the heart all the way through to the back. Because of their unique location and ability to see the backside of the heart, V_1 and V_2 are in an ideal location to diagnose posterior wall infarctions on the left ventricular side.

Acute posterior wall myocardial infarctions are seen as ST segment **depression** with **upright T waves** in leads V_1 and V_2. What? You thought acute transmural infarcts manifested as ST segment elevation! Are we crazy, or do we have short memories? No! The best way to visualize this is to imagine an inverted mirror image of an anteroseptal myocardial infarction, in which the ST segment is elevated and the T wave is inverted in V_1 and V_2. The posterior wall of the heart is right behind the anterior wall and seen by V$_1$ and V$_2$. Whatever happens on the backside of the heart is seen in reverse.

If you have a patient with a posterior wall myocardial infarction, look in leads V$_1$ and V$_2$ for ST segment depression, not elevation. This ST segment depression is also associated with an upright T wave. This is the hallmark for posterior wall myocardial infarctions. Having trouble? Just keep reading—we'll make it easier for you.

If you find it difficult to remember what a posterior infarct looks like, then you can bet we have a much easier way to make that diagnosis. We like to show you the harder way first so that the easier way will seem simpler. It's like having to tell your parents you flunked a test. You don't just walk in there and say, "Hey, Dad. Great news! I flunked my science test." No, you say something like, "Dad, I just wanted you to know before someone else told you that I wrecked the car. The friend riding with me will live, but might be in the hospital for a week or so. They don't expect his medical expenses to exceed a hundred thousand dollars. By the way, I was drunk, and the police should be here any minute." Then pause and say, "Just kidding! But I did flunk my science test." That approach makes your flunking of the science test more palatable.

Now, here's the easier way to diagnose posterior wall infarcts. Look in V$_1$ and V$_2$ and flip the EKG over by grabbing the bottom and flipping it backward so the bottom is now the top. In other words, do it vertically, not horizontally. After this, look through it from the back side, upside down. You will need a little light behind it to see through it adequately. If you do this, you will see ST segment elevation and inverted T waves in leads V$_1$ and V$_2$. This will look just like an acute anterior infarct on an upside down and backward EKG. This is a neat little trick that will stun and amaze your friends. We must confess that we did not come up with this method; it was taught to us by numerous people.

Look at the EKG in figure 92, which demonstrates an acute posterior wall myocardial infarction. *Note: Posterior wall myocardial infarctions can occur alone, but they often occur in conjunction with inferior and sometimes lateral wall myocardial infarctions.* If a patient presents with an acute inferior or lateral wall myocardial infarction, look in leads V$_1$ and V$_2$ for evidence of posterior wall involvement. Also, if a patient has a posterior infarct, don't forget to look for evidence of more extensive involvement, particularly inferiorly and laterally.

Figure 92. Example of an acute posterior and inferior infarct occurring simultaneously. Note the ST segment depression and upright T wave in V_2. Also, see the inferior ST segment elevation.

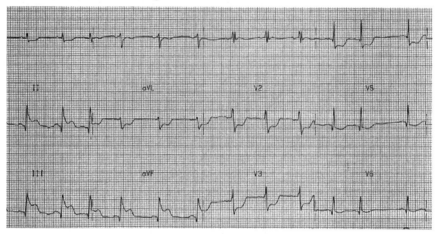

So this EKG shows us an acute posterior infarct in concert with an impressive inferior myocardial infarction. These are occurring at the same time. This can happen because the left circumflex coronary artery which feeds the posterior wall of the heart often travels farther inferiorly and feeds the inferior wall as well. Any interruption of blood flow proximally in this coronary artery will result in damage to the heart in both locations. We dare you to tear this page out of the book and flip this EKG over and look from the backside upside down. If you do, you will see what appears to be an acute anteroseptal infarction, but it would be easier just to photocopy it and do the same thing.

Electrocardiographically Silent Myocardial Infarctions

Sometimes, patients having a heart attack can have normal or near-normal-appearing EKGs. This is a potentially disturbing circumstance, especially if you have the misfortune of being an emergency room physician seeing a patient who is potentially having a heart attack. The last thing you want to do as a physician is tell a patient that there is no way he could be having a heart attack only to find out later that he died at home shortly after you discharged him. Believe us, this tragic circumstance has happened to far too many people.

Such an unfortunate tragedy is most likely to occur when the left circumflex coronary artery is the culprit causing the heart attack. The area of the heart supplied by the circumflex is historically considered an electrocardiographic "blind spot." We bring this up to warn you that **you cannot rule out a myocardial infarction in a patient with a normal EKG.** We have seen patients with myocardial infarctions who have had completely normal or almost normal electrocardiograms. Please do not forget this point when you are seeing patients in the emergency room. See the example in figure 93 of a patient who had a previous anterolateral infarct and presented with chest pain and had another infarct. Further inspection shows that the new EKG changes aren't very apparent.

Figure 93. EKG example of acute myocardial infarction with little or no gross ST segment elevation. There is a little, but not much.

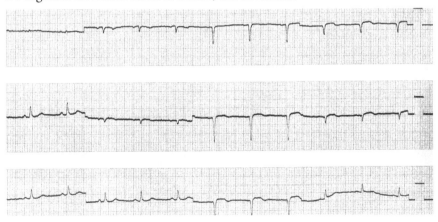

This patient has had an old anteroseptal infarct, but he also had an acute lateral infarct. The ST segment elevation is subtle and would be easy to overlook, while the old anteroseptal infarct is readily obvious.

Old Myocardial Infarctions

Old myocardial infarctions, if they were severe or large enough to damage a heart muscle, earn themselves the term **transmural** infarcts. They are called transmural because the damage extends the full thickness of the heart muscle. This means that the damage extends all the way through from the endocardium (inside) to the epicardium (outside). Most ST elevation infarcts (also called STEMIs), if not treated quickly, will result in significant heart muscle damage and will ultimately be referred to as transmural infarcts.

EKG evidence that a prior transmural myocardial infarction has occurred is manifested by the presence of **Q waves** in certain EKG leads. Now, you need to recall what a Q wave is. It is an initial downward deflection of the QRS complex. It is no more complicated than that.

It is normal to have a Q wave in some leads; however, if there are pathologic Q waves, a previous myocardial infarction (with associated scarring of the left ventricle) has occurred. For a Q wave to really mean something bad, it should be at least one little block wide and one little block deep as far as size is concerned. (Who says size doesn't matter?) As you might expect and if you are astute, Q waves are normal in the "oddball" lead AVR. Q waves can also sometimes be seen in lead III without any pathological consequence.

The location of the Q waves determines which area of the heart has been damaged. For example, Q waves in leads II, III, and AVF indicate the presence of an old inferior wall myocardial infarction. Q waves in leads V_5 and V_6 reveal the presence of an old anterolateral wall myocardial infarction. By now it should not surprise you that the rat model will confirm this yet again! Refer to your rat as you review the examples of the various infarction examples in figures 94 and 95.

Be advised that just as in a football game, where you might have offsetting penalties, it is entirely possible to have multiple myocardial infarctions that could offset one another—at least as far as the EKG is concerned. We don't mean to imply that they offset so that the patient is fine. We do mean, however, that multiple areas of damage can affect the EKG in such a way as to cancel each other out, in effect erasing Q waves. For example, a patient with a preexisting inferior wall myocardial infarction who has had another infarct that affects the anterior wall might erase the Q waves that were present in the inferior wall. The reverse can happen, as well. The point to remember is that an absence of Q waves does not necessarily rule out a previous myocardial infarction. This is simply one more example of why computers will never replace humans when it comes to interpreting EKGs.

Figure 94. Old inferior infarct: note inferior Q waves in leads II, III, and AVF. They're small, but they're there.

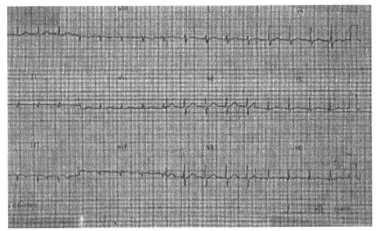

Looking closely at the EKG above, you will notice one more interesting thing about its appearance. This won't be hard to figure out if you really think about it. Go ahead and look at it again and compare it to the other EKGs you've seen thus far. Okay, so you don't quite get it? That's all right. We are going to tell you. Look at the overall size of the QRS complexes. Do you notice that the voltage is lower? It is because two parts of this patient's heart muscle are missing. Part of the anterior wall and part of the inferior wall are gone. This dead heart tissue can no longer contribute to the electrical energy that generates the QRS complex as the heart contracts; therefore, the QRS complexes have to be smaller. Noting this odd low voltage and looking at an old EKG are clues of what has really happened to this patient.

Figure 95. Old anterior-septal infarct with anterior Q waves.

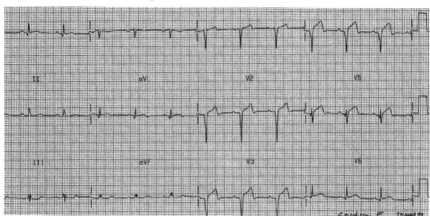

Beware of Q waves in leads V_1, V_2, and V_3. Their presence might represent an old anteroseptal myocardial infarction but could also be because of inappropriate lead placement. If in doubt, have the technician move the V leads down an interspace on the patient's chest and repeat the EKG. If the patient has had a previous anteroseptal myocardial infarction, then the Q waves will remain in these leads. If it's because of lead placement, then the Q waves will change to R waves in these leads.

This reminds us of our **EKG third commandment**: *Beware of the treacherous technician.* Also, a LAFB might cause the occurrence of Q waves in leads V_1 and V_2, while a left posterior fascicular block might cause Q waves to be present in the inferior leads. Sorry, you just might have to memorize those facts.

Left Bundle Branch Block and Myocardial Infarctions

If you are a very experienced electrocardiographer, it is possible to read acute myocardial infarctions through a left bundle branch block. Unfortunately, space does not allow a dissertation on this, and we want you to focus on the fundamentals for now, so we will not address this topic other than to say that you really need an old EKG for a point of reference, and you have to look very carefully at the ST segments for evidence of elevation. This can be a tall task as it is hard to discriminate where the QRS complex ends and the ST segment begins in a patient that has a LBBB.

Right Bundle Branch Block and Myocardial Infarctions

It is much easier to read an old, or completed, myocardial infarction through a right bundle branch block than a left bundle branch block. An old myocardial infarction, as you recall, often causes the EKG to develop Q waves in leads that reflect where the damage has occurred. Because the RBBB affects only the terminal portion of the QRS complex and not the start of it, you would expect that in an instance of an old myocardial infarction with coexisting RBBB, the Q waves that previously formed (as a result of the old infarct) would persist—and they do. Not only do they remain, they are easy to see if you look for them.

It may be difficult to interpret an EKG with RBBB and an acute myocardial infarction. This is because the RBBB will obscure the beginning of the ST segment. Remember that **the ST segment is elevated in acute transmural myocardial infarction**. The presence of the RBBB affects the end of the QRS, which makes accurate interpretation of what the ST segment is doing a little dicey. To get around this, you have to visually remove the RBBB portion from the terminal portion of the QRS; you can then analyze the ST segment for displacement. If the ST segment is elevated, after allowing for the terminal portion of the QRS to be abnormal from the RBBB, then you can accurately interpret acute myocardial infarctions through a RBBB. See figure 96.

Figure 96. Example of acute posterolateral infarction with an underlying RBBB: note the slightly elevated ST segments in leads I and AVL and the depressed ST segments in leads V$_1$ and V$_2$.

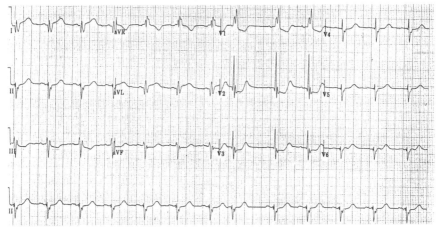

The preceding is a difficult one, to say the least. The authors might have missed this one in a stack of many to read. You are learning more than you realize now.

This concludes our section on myocardial infarctions, both acute and old. We want to leave you with the thought that myocardial infarctions can be electrocardiographically silent, so you might want to be on the alert for this. This will require you—the physician or monitor technician—to be vigilant. It never hurts to listen to the patient's history when you interpret a diagnostic test. You also need to be mindful of pericarditis and aneurysms masquerading as an acute myocardial infarction. And lastly, don't forget about early repolarization changes, which are notorious for mimicking acute myocardial infarctions. Early repolarization is pervasive in young black men in particular.

If moonlighting in the emergency room and handed an EKG that appears to reveal an acute myocardial infarction, remember the fourth EKG commandment, which states: "Thou shall not attempt to interpret an EKG without looking at the patient's prior tracings." It's amazing how helpful it can be to have an old EKG for comparison to determine whether or not the ST segment elevation you see is because of an acute myocardial infarction or another cause.

CHAPTER 7: PACED BEATS AND PACED RHYTHMS

This is a perfect time to introduce implantable cardiac pacemakers. We'll have a brief review of pacemaker nomenclature, then give you examples of various paced cardiac rhythms. But as usual, let's put the subject into some real-life context by talking about who might benefit from a pacemaker and why.

Pacemakers are implanted because of some abnormality in the heart's native electrical system. The most common problem necessitating pacemaker implantation is when the sinus node fatigues or is damaged and fails to set an electrical tempo.

Because the heart won't beat unless it receives an electrical impulse, a failing sinoatrial node (called the pacemaker of the heart) will result in a very slow or even absent heartbeat.

The sinoatrial node can, and often does, malfunction as a result of aging alone. It can also be effected by diseases, such as sarcoidosis and myocarditis. Prior infarcts can also damage the sinoatrial node, inhibiting its normal function, which is, as you already know, to pace the heart rhythmically.

Farther on down the conduction system, there exists a backup system of pacemaking for the heart should the SA node fail to perform its job. Next in the chain of command is the AV node. If the sinus node fails, usually the AV node will notice this and take over. When the AV node is responsible for setting the pacing rate, it does so at a much slower rate than the sinoatrial node.

Rhythms that originate within the AV node are defined as **junctional** or **nodal rhythms**. Rhythms that have their origin in one of the ventricles are called **ventricular rhythms**.

Lastly, there can be conduction blocks in the bundle of His and farther downstream in the right and left bundle branches. Regardless of the cause, a pathologically slow heart rate can be overcome by implanting a permanent pacemaker. The pacemaker can be programmed at whatever minimal rate the physician decides is appropriate for the patient.

Pacemakers are spoken of in terms of a nomenclature system that has been accepted worldwide. This nomenclature system allows physicians in one country to speak to physicians in another country and understand one another. Sounds silly, but it's necessary.

It's customary that pacemakers are identified by a system of sequential letters. The letters designate what type of pacemaker is present. This designation depends on several key issues. The characteristics of the implanted pacemaker determine how we refer to and name that pacemaker. The nomenclature for pacemakers answers the following questions: Which chamber is the pacer pacing? Which chamber is the pacer sensing? What mode of action does the pacer use to pace? Are there any special features of the pacemaker that make it unique or work better? The answers to these questions are revealed in the aforementioned letter abbreviation format.

It isn't our intent to get into any great detail here; however, a basic understanding of pacemaker nomenclature is important. The **first** letter in pacemaker nomenclature denotes the **chamber paced**. That is simple enough. There are only two chambers to pace, the atrium or the ventricle. If it were the ventricle and only the ventricle being paced, then a **V** would be the appropriate first letter in the nomenclature system. If it were the atrium being paced, then an **A** would be the appropriate letter. If it were true that **both** chambers (i.e., the atrium and the ventricle being paced) were being paced, then a **D** would be written. The **D** designation indicates that is a **dual**-chamber pacemaker.

Reread that. It is not very complicated. Three letters so far and all the letters make logical sense.

The **second** letter in the nomenclature system indicates the chamber sensed. By sensing, we mean that in order for a pacer to know when to pace, it has to know when the native rhythm is working as expected. To accomplish this, the pacemaker can't simply send out electrical stimuli to generate a heartbeat indiscriminately; rather, it has to be capable of detecting a native heartbeat. You wouldn't want a pacemaker implanted in you that fired all the time regardless of your own intrinsic rhythm. Not only would it be a waste of perfectly good energy, but it might kill you as well. The pacemaker's ability to detect a natural heartbeat is what we refer to as sensing. So the second letter in the nomenclature system is reserved for the chamber the pacemaker is sensing. If it were the atria, then an **A** would be appropriate. If it were the ventricle, then a **V** would be appropriate. If it were both the atria and ventricle sensed, then a **D** would be appropriate the letter—indicating dual-chamber sensing. Do you see a pattern here?

The **third** letter in the nomenclature system indicates the mode of functioning of the pacemaker. This indicates whether the pacemaker is **triggered** by an electrical event, or **inhibited** by an electrical event, or both. If it is triggered, a **T** goes in the third location. If it's inhibited, it's an **I**. And if it's triggered and inhibited, a **D** is the appropriate letter in that location. As you have guessed, D means dual.

The **fourth** and final letter in the nomenclature system indicates what special properties the pacemaker has, such as **rate responsive modes**. If it has a rate responsive mode, then an **R** would be located here. If it has no special feature, then no letter will be placed, and it will be only a three-letter designation. That is a very concise but complete summary of how pacemakers are described.

After reading a technical section, you need to have the points driven into your brain. We'll do this through the use of examples, and you'll be glad we congealed everything for you.

A simple pacemaker is a ventricular single chamber pacemaker. In this primitive example, the pacemaker is inhibited as its mode of functioning. The universal designation for this pacemaker would then be **VVI**. In this circumstance, there is one lead implanted in the patient and attached to the generator. This single lead is placed and secured inside the apex (or tip) of the right ventricle. From here, the pacer can fire and activate the right ventricle when necessary to produce a much-needed heartbeat. It also can sense any remaining electrical activity the right ventricle might produce on its own. If it senses a native heartbeat, it will inhibit itself from firing so it does not compete with the native rhythm. And just to fill you in completely, people who have pacers often only need pacing some of the time. In other words, rarely is a patient totally pacer dependent. Sometimes, the patient needs the pacer to fire to keep a regular and consistent heartbeat while at other times, the patient's natural rhythm works just fine.

An example of a more complicated pacemaker would be a dual-chamber device. In this case, there are two leads, one in the right atrium and one in the right ventricle. Because in this situation there are two leads, it won't surprise you that we designate it as a **DDD** pacer. Incidentally, the third D indicates that the pacer is triggered and inhibited, as most dual-chamber pacers are. A dual-chamber pacemaker that has a rate responsive mode would be designated as a **DDDR** pacer. It isn't necessary to pursue this discussion any farther as long as you have a basic understanding of pacemaker nomenclature.

Now you have all the information you need to read paced EKGs.

Paced Beats

We are going to illustrate for you, through various examples, how to interpret paced EKGs. Just follow along. It stands to reason that a dual-chamber pacemaker can pace either in the atrium, the ventricle, or both. An atrial-paced beat will appear as a pacer spike preceding a P wave. You will see that the P wave morphology (or appearance and shape) will be different from the usual appearing sinus node generated P wave. The paced P wave morphology, however, will be consistent from beat to beat. See figure 97.

Figure 97. Atrial-paced beats: see the large atrial pacer spikes preceding each QRS complex.

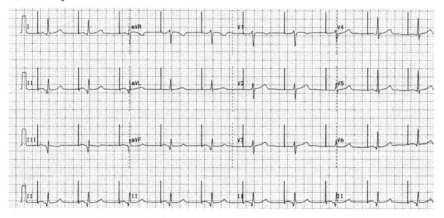

This pacer has a **unipolar lead** as opposed to a **bipolar lead**. Unipolar leads leave large pacer spikes, whereas bipolar leads leave small pacer spikes that might be difficult to see. You won't run across too many unipolar leads, so prepare yourself to look carefully for atrial pacer spikes.

Atrial Sensing with Ventricular Pacing

When a dual-chamber pacemaker is implanted in a patient with a functioning sinus node (where the atrial activity is intact), but who has impaired or blocked AV conduction, it'll be necessary for the pacer to sense the atrial activity first and then create an electrical bridge to the ventricles. Again, the pacer does not want to compete with the SA node, so it must inhibit itself from pacing there. The pacer will, once it detects an atrial beat, wait patiently for the right ventricle to fire on its own. The right ventricular lead will be responsible for looking for the timely occurrence of the impending ventricular beat. If it does not sense a ventricular beat within a predetermined time frame, it will pace on the ventricular side of the heart. It paces only if the right ventricle fails to fire on its own after a sensed atrial event. This will result in the dual-chamber pacer sensing the atrial activity and pacing only on the ventricular side. In this hypothetical case, there'll be an absence of atrial pacer spikes because of the presence of a native P wave. The P waves, however, will be followed by paced ventricular beats. See figure 98.

Figure 98. Example of atrial sensing and ventricular pacing: this must be a DDD pacer then. Note the normal P wave and the paced QRS beats following each sinus P wave.

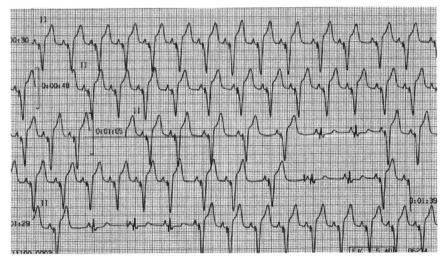

Notice the native P waves followed by the wide QRS complexes. These wide QRS complexes are paced ventricular beats. If you look carefully, you can see the small pacer spikes preceding each widened QRS (see fig. 99).

Figure 99. 12-lead example of AV pacing where both the atria and ventricle are paced. Note atrial and ventricular pacer spikes.

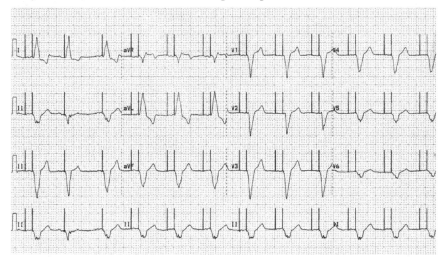

Notice the very prominent unipolar pacer spikes that are pretty close together. These are atrial and ventricular pacer spikes. The P waves following the atrial pacer spikes are small and hard to see. If you look closely at the left side of the EKG in lead I, you will see a native P wave and just one ventricular pacer spike. This pacer appropriately inhibited pacing on the atrial side when it sensed a native P wave.

Asynchronous Ventricular Pacing

When pacemakers first came into being, they were simple. They were all one-lead systems—just a ventricular lead with no lead in the atrium. Primitive is a better way to put it. This type of pacer has no way of sensing what electrical events are happening in the atria. In this setting, ventricular pacemakers will fire without regard to atrial activity. That's a bad thing because there is no conservation of AV synchrony. Recalling physiology, the atria contract first, followed by the ventricles. Any deviation from this sequence is fraught with peril.

In figures 100 and 101, note that the P waves occur spontaneously and regularly, while the ventricular pacemaker fires at a constant rate. This happens regardless of native atrial beats. This is how pacemakers functioned in the early days before we learned that this scenario could lead to **pacemaker syndrome**. Pacemaker syndrome is the term used for the very uncomfortable feeling patients get when they have asynchronous pacing. More advanced technology has allowed us to maintain AV synchrony and simultaneously retain normal hemodynamic function. This can be accomplished only with dual-chamber sensing and pacing.

Can you think of a clinical scenario in which a single ventricular lead pacemaker would be appropriate? Think hard. How about atrial fibrillation with a very slow ventricular response? There would be no use for an atrial lead, because the atrial fibrillation doesn't generate enough electricity for the pacer to sense. Not only that, but the fibrillating atrium can't be paced anyway.

Figure 100. Example of asynchronous ventricular pacing.

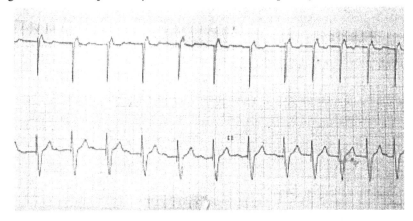

Figure 101. Ventricular pacing without regard to P waves.

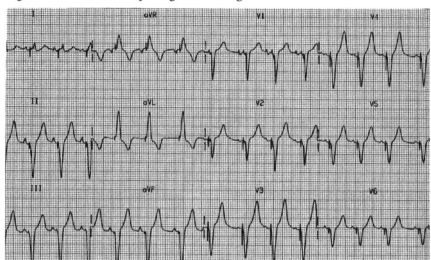

The two above examples are similar in that both result in loss of AV synchrony. It's important to maintain AV synchrony if at all possible. If you were the patient and needed a pacemaker, you wouldn't care for the way you felt if that didn't happen. Pacemaker syndrome is quite uncomfortable. Not only is the loss of AV synchrony uncomfortable, it puts excessive pressure on the upper chambers of the heart causing them to enlarge, and that's not a good thing either.

A physician once told us, "When you put in a pacemaker, three things can happen, and two of them are bad." That is a short but accurate statement. We need to mention a couple of things that can go wrong when pacemakers are implanted.

The first undesirable outcome is the potential for the pacer to fail to do its job, and that is pace the heart. If the pacer doesn't pace, then you didn't do the patient any favors by putting it in—that's obvious. This problem is also referred to as failure to capture. If the pacer generator sends out an electrical stimulus that fails to elicit a QRS complex, then this is failure to capture. This type of pacer malfunction can result from lead dislodgement, scarring in the heart, or lead fracture. This will be revealed on an EKG as the appearance of a pacer spike that isn't followed by a P wave or a QRS complex. Just so you will know, failure to pace can occur on the atrial side or the ventricular side. If it happens only in the atria, then a P wave will not follow an atrial pacer spike. A similar circumstance occurs when the ventricular lead fails to capture, and the ventricular pacer spikes are not followed by QRS complexes. You guessed it. If everything goes wrong—and sometimes medicine and interventions do follow Murphy's law—you can be sure that both leads could fail, and all you might see are atrial and ventricular pacer spikes with no P waves or QRS complexes. In that circumstance, you had better be quick to remedy the problem or it might not matter long because if the patient is pacer dependent, then he will be dead real soon.

Another problem we have seen with pacemakers is **pacer malsensing**. This means that the pacer is unable to sense either native atrial or ventricular beats or even both in worst-case scenarios. If this occurs, you might see pacer spikes attempting to pace at inappropriate times. This is dangerous and needs immediate correction. The causes for this are the same as above or could be a problem with programming of the generator.

We need to mention **pacemaker mediated tachycardia** (PMT). This is what we call an iatrogenic problem—one that the treatment, namely, implantation of the device, caused. This occurs because of a programming error with the pacemaker itself and an ill-timed early heartbeat to set the process in motion. The pacemaker generator can be fooled into pacing too fast because of a combination of sensing errors and other variables being out of adjustment. If you think a patient with a pacemaker is having PMT, place a magnet over the pacer generator. This will cause the pacer to pace at a fixed rate regardless of the intrinsic rhythm of the patient's heart. The magnet turns the sensing function of the pacer off. If it is PMT, then the problem will immediately resolve. PMT usually ticks along at well over one hundred beats a minute with no obvious provocation. It is usually happens when the pacer gets confused. The device believes it is recognizing atrial tachycardia and following it on the ventricular side with no beat to beat variability. In effect, the pacer "thinks" the atria are beating fast, therefore it should pace the ventricles at the same rate. Of course, in PMT, that is not really happening; the pacemaker just thinks it is, so it does what it is programmed to do. To avoid this, the PVARP (or **post-ventricular atrial refractory period**) has to be extended. But this is something a competent pacer rep will recognize and do for you if asked.

We believe that's all you really need to know about pacemakers and how to interpret the EKGs done on patients who have them. Be aware that it can get much more complicated than what we have illustrated, but you are on your way to continuing to expand your fund of knowledge.

CHAPTER 8: ELECTROLYTES AND THE HEART

Patients have some catchy and unique ways of describing what's wrong with them. We've heard patients with cirrhosis of the liver refer to their condition as "roaches of the liver." We've also had patients refer to electrolyte abnormalities in their blood as "electric light" abnormalities. We are now going to discuss "electric light" abnormalities and their potential effect on the EKG.

Because the heart's function is highly dependent on electrolyte concentration gradients across the cell membranes that make up the heart muscle, it should be apparent that abnormal electrolyte concentrations in the blood can cause some pretty interesting abnormalities.

Boneheads, relax! This isn't going to stress you too much, because we are only talking about three little electrolytes here: **potassium**, **calcium**, and **magnesium**. We'll look at what effects elevated and reduced levels of these ions have on the EKG.

As you might recall from biochemistry, the electrical gradient across the myocardial cell membrane is generated by the activity of the **electrogenic sodium potassium pump**. This pump, which removes three sodium ions from the cell while putting two potassium ions into the cell per pump cycle, leaves the inside of the cell relative to the outside deficient in one positive charge. Think about it. If you take three positive charges out of something and put two back in, then there will be a net loss of one positive charge inside the cell each time the pump functions. This electrogenic pump then renders the inside of the cell negative relative to the outside of the cell. This is the process that generates the **resting negative membrane potential**. This membrane potential is also generated by the sequestration of anions (negatively charged particles) within the cell. The heart muscle cells must maintain a net negative charge of about 90 millivolts to function.

The cells of the heart must have a resting negative membrane potential in order for an action potential to occur. It is the action potential that causes the heart to beat. The heart couldn't be triggered to beat without being negatively charged first. Again, this negative resting membrane potential has been measured by professionals who analyze such things to be in the realm of minus 90 millivolts. Normal physiology requires that the concentration of sodium inside the cell be much lower than the sodium concentration outside of the cell. The reverse is true for potassium. It is these ion concentration gradients, which generate the electrical difference across the cell membrane, that allow an action potential to occur. It's easy to fathom that abnormalities in ion concentration gradients have the potential to alter the resting membrane potential. The altered membrane potential will adversely affect depolarization and repolarization, which will be reflected on the EKG.

Hypokalemia

Let's review potassium first. Serum potassium levels can be high or low, and either situation can be potentially harmful and even fatal if untreated. **Hypokalemia**, which is a low blood serum potassium level, can be brought about by several things, including diuretic use, vomiting, renal potassium wasting diseases, hyperaldosteronism, and other diseases. When hypokalemia is suspected, the EKG can assist in making the diagnosis (though with the readily available lab testing, a serum potassium level is the most appropriate way to make the diagnosis). It is amazing, when you think about it, that you can make the diagnosis of hypokalemia just by looking at an EKG. When you have the knowledge to do this, you can astound your fellow students. So what are the EKG manifestations of hypokalemia? In addition to increased myocardial electrical irritability, which can result in any number of arrhythmias (e.g., PVCs and ventricular tachycardia, PACs, atrial flutter and atrial fibrillation), hypokalemia has effects on the U waves, ST segments, T waves, and QT interval. Yes, you have to know and understand all of these, so let's get started.

One very important EKG manifestation of hypokalemia includes the presence of prominent **U waves**. We don't talk about U waves much, so this is a somewhat rare instance where U waves are really important. Recall that the U waves occur at the end of the T waves and are often unnoticeable. As the hypokalemia progresses, the T waves become smaller and the U waves become larger. So when you think of hypokalemia, think of large U waves and small T waves. You can remember that; if not, write it down. Often, you can't really see the U waves on an EKG unless hypokalemia is present, so their appearance should make you at least curious. What else occurs when a patient has low potassium? Keep reading.

The **ST segment** will likely become mildly **depressed**. That's not all. In extreme cases of hypokalemia, **T wave inversion** occurs as well. Normally upright T waves flip right over and become negative. Hypokalemia also causes the appearance of a **long Q-T interval**. We have already mentioned that a long QT is associated with potentially lethal arrhythmias such as **Torsades de pointes**. In the case of hypokalemia, the QT prolongation occurs not as a result of lengthening of the time interval from the beginning of the QRS to the end of the T wave but rather because of the addition of the prominent U wave at the end of the T wave. Read that again for clarity and think about it for a minute. This addition of the U wave causes the T wave to appear fatter than usual, making the QT interval appear longer. We call this a **long QT-U interval**, if you want to be really specific. Note the examples of hypokalemia in figure 102. The EKG manifestations readily revert when the potassium is repleted.

The treatment of hypokalemia is simple. Replace it!

Figure 102. EKG example of hypokalemia: note the very prominent U waves circled and the relatively small T waves. The QT-U interval is also lengthened.

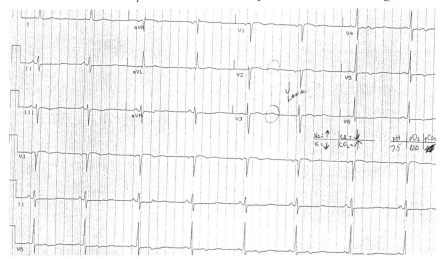

Hyperkalemia

This electrolyte abnormality, which is an elevated potassium level, is often seen in patients with **chronic renal insufficiency** or **acute renal failure**. It also occurs in patients who are taking potassium supplements and those who are on potassium-sparing diuretics, such as spironolactone. Patients who are prescribed angiotensin-converting enzyme inhibitors and angiotensin receptor blockers might also develop hyperkalemia. The heart is very sensitive to hyperkalemia, and it will let you know it with EKG abnormalities and arrhythmias.

The most striking and frequent EKG manifestations of hyperkalemia are the **T waves** becoming **peaked** and pinching at the base (see fig. 103). Normally, when you look at an EKG and compare the overall amplitude of the QRS complexes to that of the T waves, the T wave's amplitude (or height) will measure about a third that of the QRS complexes. In hyperkalemia, the T waves can be half as tall as the QRSs or even taller. The T waves are not the only things affected. The **P waves** become **small,** and if the situation gets bad enough they might eventually disappear altogether. Thought we were through? Not yet. The **PR intervals** can **lengthen.** As the hyperkalemia progresses, the ST segments become depressed and the **QRS duration lengthens**, giving the QRSs a wider appearance. If the QRS widens too much, an untimely death can occur as a consequence of **ventricular fibrillation**. If you don't know it, ventricular fibrillation is a life-ending arrhythmia—if not immediately corrected with a strong jolt of electricity (a procedure called a cardioversion). So, if you have a patient with hyperkalemia and you see EKG evidence supporting that assessment, then act quickly to correct the problem. It's best to put a patient with hyperkalemia in a monitored bed as soon as possible, because life-threatening arrhythmias can occur abruptly and unpredictably.

Again, we need to tell you the treatment. You have options here. The first option is to give the patient intravenous calcium. The second option is to give insulin and glucose at the same time. This combination will drive the serum potassium into the cell, thereby lowering the blood potassium level.

Figure 103. Example of hyperkalemia: note the peaked and pinched T waves.

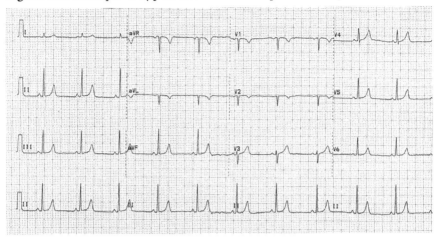

At the outset of this book we promised to teach you how to read EKGs, and we hope we are doing a good job of it. Now let's integrate your knowledge of EKG reading and apply it to a practical situation that you'll likely encounter. After all, isn't that the reason anyone studies a subject, to apply the knowledge to reap some benefit? To that end, if you have a patient with EKG changes that are consistent with severe hyperkalemia, then get that patient to a monitored bed immediately. Waiting to treat the hyperkalemia or confirm its presence with another blood test could result in the patient's death. This is a tough lesson to learn the hard way. Learn it now!

Calcium

Hypocalcemia, which is a low serum calcium level, is not common. If you're around long enough, you'll see it. Hypocalcemia causes the QT interval to increase. This prolongation of the QT interval is actually prolongation of the QT interval as measured from the **beginning of the QRS to the beginning of the T wave**. Now, that might sound a little picky. Why are we making such a big deal out of how the QT is prolonged? Because we want you to remember that hypokalemia caused QT prolongation as well. But QT prolongation in hypokalemia is unique in that it prolongs the interval by adding a fat U wave to the end of the T wave. The appearance of QT prolongation on the EKG from hypocalcemia is different from that of hypokalemia. Yes, you have to know both—sorry. So know that **in hypocalcemia, the Q to the onset of the T wave is lengthened**. See figure 104.

Figure 104. EKG example of hypocalcemia: note the long QT interval.

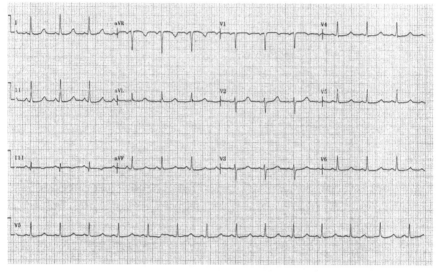

Hypercalcemia

Hypercalcemia (an elevated serum calcium level) is manifested as the reverse of hypocalcemia. In this circumstance, the QT interval is **shortened**. And again, this shortening occurs primarily from the end of the QRS to the beginning of the T wave. The T wave itself is not short. So, the Q to the onset of the T wave is shortened in hypercalcemia. See figure 105. We once had a patient with **multiple myeloma** who was markedly hypercalcemic, and we made the diagnosis from the EKG alone.

Figure 105. EKG example of hypercalcemia: note the short QT interval. The T wave appears jammed-up on the QRS.

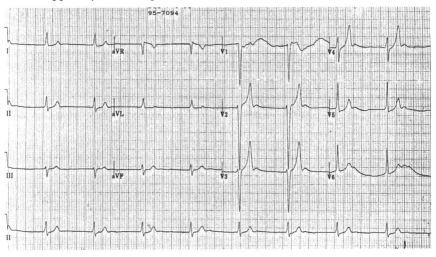

Magnesium

Just as calcium and potassium levels can be high or low, so can magnesium levels. Unfortunately, abnormal levels of serum magnesium are mostly electrocardiographically stealth, that is until a life-threatening arrhythmia occurs. When an EKG abnormality is apparent with hypomagnesemia, it is QT interval prolongation. We concern ourselves so much with the length of the QT interval because it initiates the malicious arrhythmia called **Torsades de pointes**. The more you see it, the more you'll see why it is called that. Note the example of hypomagnesemia in figure 106 that resulted in Torsades de pointes.

Figure 106. Rhythm strip example of hypomagnesemia resulting in Torsades de pointes.

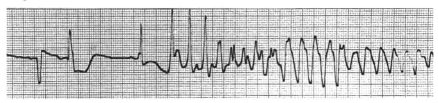

That is about all you really need to know about electrolyte abnormalities and the heart. Mind you, there are others, and we could go on, but delving further into the subject just runs the risk of confusing you. If you are a physician or plan to become one, we want you to be aware that slight alterations in blood chemistry levels can have dramatic and potentially fatal results. If as a physician you are treating a patient's hypertension with a diuretic, remember that diuretics can cause the kidneys to lose potassium. You will want to check the serum potassium level on them shortly after starting the diuretic so that you can correct the hypokalemia before something bad happens. It does the patient little good to have his blood pressure fixed only to be found dead on the sidewalk a few days later from an iatrogenically induced arrhythmia.

Be advised also that some of the drugs you prescribe also can affect the QT interval as an unintended side effect. Learn those that do and make an effort to remember them. If you don't know if the drug you are prescribing to a patient has the potential to prolong the QT interval, then look it up. You would seldom ever want to combine two QT prolonging drugs in one patient. When you have to put a patient on a medicine that prolongs the QT interval, you had better measure it. If the QT interval gets too long from the medicine, then the risk of the medicine isn't worth the benefit.

CHAPTER 9: MISCELLANEOUS CONDITIONS

There are abnormalities on the EKG that don't really fit into any of the categories already discussed. There are also diseases and clinical conditions for that matter that exist that need to be mentioned. We would like to review some of those with you. Some of them are common and others are rare, but we feel that your education would be incomplete if we didn't mention them. We will discuss more esoteric abnormalities in the test-tracing section at the end. We do hope you are enjoying yourself.

Pericarditis

Pericarditis is a common abnormality that we guarantee you will see in your clinical experience. Recall that this is a condition in which the pericardial sac (the friction-relieving sac surrounding the heart) becomes inflamed. The inflammation can be caused by infectious agents such as viruses and bacteria. It can also result from an abnormal immunologic response like those seen in patients afflicted with rheumatoid arthritis and **systemic lupus erythematosus** (SLE). More often, it is idiopathic, which means "we aren't smart enough to figure out why it occurs." Regardless of the cause, pericarditis *hurts*! Patients with pericarditis complain of sharp pain in the center of their chest. This intense pain gets worse when they lie on their backs. The pain universally eases some when they sit up. Remember this! If you have a stethoscope at your disposal, use it to listen to their chest wall. If you do this, you'll often hear a to-and-fro friction rub in patients who have pericarditis. Yes, that's right! A to-and-fro friction rub. What is that you wonder? It sounds a lot like a washing machine running. Imagine that, a patient's body sounding like a kitchen appliance.

Not only does pericarditis hurt, but it can cause some interesting and harmful hemodynamic problems. Imagine the heart sitting in a relatively slick but only mildly compliant sac. Inflammation occurs that can result from an immune response. Before you know it, the pericardial sac is filled with unwanted things, such as white blood cells, blood, and serous fluid. Now the heart is physically bound and is unable to fill because there's no expansion space. During diastole (the heart's relaxation phase), the heart must be free to fill with blood before it can pump the blood back out to the body. Since blood is constantly returning to the heart from the body and has to have some place to go, the backup of blood that can't be accommodated by the hard-to-fill heart will be seen as **jugular venous distention**, or JVD for short. If the process worsens, the cardiac output will drop so low as to affect the blood pressure, and the patient will eventually lose consciousness—or even die. In this setting, an emergency procedure called a **pericardiocentesis** must be performed to remove the offending fluid. There is nothing more rewarding to a doctor than to treat a patient who has one foot in a coffin and the other on a banana peel by sticking a needle into his pericardial sac and extracting blood and fluid so that his heart can resume its normal function, allowing the patient to go on living another day.

Figure 107. EKG example of pericarditis with global ST segment elevation and PR segment depression in all leads, except for AVR.

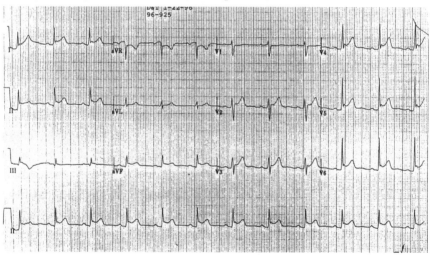

The key with this one is to see the ST segment elevation and then notice that it is present in every lead, except AVR (see fig. 107). The next clue is that the PR segment, when carefully examined, is somewhat depressed. Recall that this differs from ST segment elevation because of a heart attack. During a heart attack, the ST segment elevation is convex and the PR segments aren't depressed.

Electrical Alternans

Electrical alternans involves a shifting of the electrical axis on the EKG with every other beat of the heart. It is commonly seen in the case of cardiac **tamponade**. Tamponade is when the pericardial sac fills with so much fluid, be it blood or other fluid, that it inhibits the heart from its normal filling process. Electrical alternans might be seen in other disorders; however, tamponade is the clinical syndrome we want you to associate with this. See the example of electrical alternans noted in figure 108. It generally indicates a hemodynamically significant **pericardial effusion** that needs immediate attention. We know you already know this; we just want to make sure. Sometimes you have to say things twice. Sometimes you have to say things twice.

Figure 108. EKG example of electrical alternans: note the obvious voltage changes every other beat.

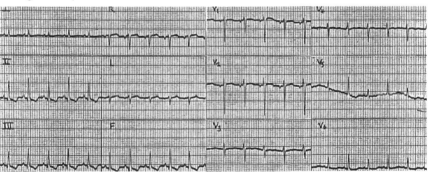

In the above example, if you look carefully, you'll see there is the occurrence of a fairly large QRS immediately followed by a smaller QRS. This process repeats itself over and over through the course of the

EKG. It's best seen in figure 108 in leads V_1 and V_2, large QRS followed by small QRS, and so on.

Dextrocardia

Dextrocardia is the clinical situation in which the heart is located on the wrong side of the chest. This scenario is a wonderful opportunity for a green medical student to make the attending physician look bad. We suspect you know that normally the heart favors the left side of the chest. In the case of dextrocardia, it's located more on the right side of the chest. To make matters worse, patients with dextrocardia often take great pleasure in making their doctors look stupid. This type of patient loves to fail to inform the poor physician of his anomaly. Some, however, come to medical attention and legitimately don't know that they were born the reverse of the rest of us. Regardless, an abnormally located heart can cause consternation on the part of the doctor interpreting the EKG. On a patient who has true dextrocardia, a standard EKG lead placement will result in the appearance of an old extensive anterolateral myocardial infarction (see fig. 109). That might come as a shock to the parent of a fourteen-year-old boy getting ready to play football. For the Bonehead, clues to the presence of dextrocardia from the EKG are beyond the scope of this book. However, if you suspect dextrocardia then reverse the chest leads and perform right-sided chest leads instead. With this procedure, R waves will become apparent in the lateral right-sided precordial leads. We also recommend just asking the patient if he has been told that his heart is on the wrong side of his chest. Most of them will "fess up."

Figure 109. EKG example of dextrocardia: note the lack of R waves in the precordial leads and the right axis deviation.

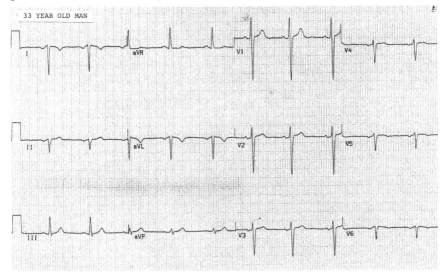

Lead Misplacement

Lead misplacement can rear its ugly head at any time and in many ways. When you see an EKG that seems to make no physiologic sense, then think whether the leads could have been inadvertently reversed. You'll be amazed to find out how often this happens. Don't let the grubby medical student or treacherous technicians make you look stupid.

Accelerated AV Conduction

Previously discussed Wolff-Parkinson-White syndrome; however, there are other routes of AV nodal bypass that leave the AV node out of the loop. As in WPW, they bypass the AV node and plug into the bundle of His. There is a syndrome known as **Lown-Ganong-Levine**, in which the P-R interval is short while the QRS remains of normal duration. No delta wave is evident as you would see with WPW. Patients with this syndrome have episodes of tachycardia very similar to those who have WPW. Note the EKG in figure 110.

Figure 110. Example of Lown-Ganong-Levine: note the short PR interval. See also that the QRS duration is normal with an absence of a delta wave or slurred upstroke of the QRS, as you would expect with Wolff-Parkinson-White syndrome.

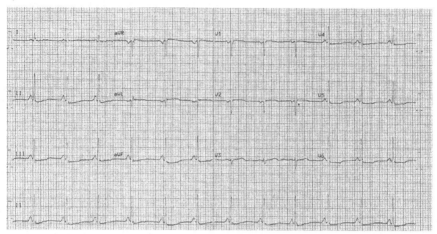

The P wave in this example is pressed right up next to the QRS. This appearance indicates that the normal AV delay is absent. This is also known as accelerated AV conduction. Patients with this anatomy are prone to rapid supraventricular arrhythmias.

Long Q-T Interval

Remember—and this is a recurring theme—that if something can be too long or too short, it must be measured. As soon as you don't measure it, it'll be abnormal. So get into the habit of measuring all the intervals we've mentioned. In the case of QT prolongation, it's helpful to have some familiarity with what causes it. Common culprits are drugs. **Class I-A antiarrhythmic drugs** (quinidine, procainamide, and disopyramide) have been notoriously associated with QT prolongation, as have electrolyte abnormalities, particularly hypomagnesemia and hypocalcemia. There are **congenital** diseases that cause prolongation of the QT interval, primarily **Romano-Ward** and **Jervell-Lange-Nielsen**. Jervell-Lange-Nielsen syndrome involves congenital **deafness** and a long Q-T interval, while Romano-Ward syndrome involves just a prolonged Q-T interval without congenital deafness. The presence of these syndromes can be a marker for sudden cardiac death. The take home here is to **measure the QT interval on all of the EKGs you read**. You can't know whether it's too long or too short if you don't take the time to measure it. It should always be less than half the preceding R-R cycle length.

Chronic Pulmonary Disease Pattern

Dr. William Nelson, during our training, spoke of **Schamroth's sign**. This EKG finding is marked by flattening of the P wave, QRS, and T wave in lead I. It is also associated with the presence of S waves in the lateral precordial leads in patients with significant lung disease. The EKG in figure 111 illustrates this fairly well.

Figure 111. 12-lead of a lung disease patient showing Schamroth's sign: note the low-voltage P, QRS, and T wave in lead I. Also see the deep S wave in V_6.

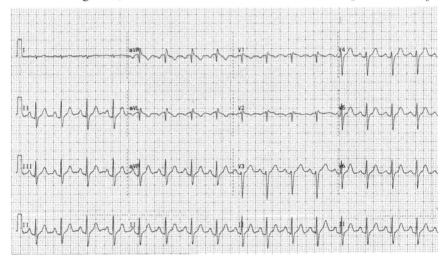

You'll want to learn this so that you can make your friends and maybe even your attending physician on rounds appear not-so-well educated. When you see an EKG with a vertical axis, barely discernible T waves, QRSs, and P waves in lead I, and the EKG was performed on a patient who is blue and very short of breath, let it be known that this patient has Schamroth's sign. Also tell them that if they look carefully, they will see an undulating baseline that is barely discernible in figure 111. Baseline undulating is the result of the patient's heavy breathing.

Hypothermia

The EKG manifestations of profound hypothermia are unique and termed **Osborne waves**, or **J waves**. We didn't coin these terms. We read them in many books. Note the example in figure 112 of a patient who was really cold. We don't think you'll see this often, but you could see it during the winter, especially if you live in some place cold that has a lot of homeless people.

Figure 112. EKG example of hypothermia: note the J wave, which is seen very well in this example in lead V_4. It occurs just at the end of the QRS.

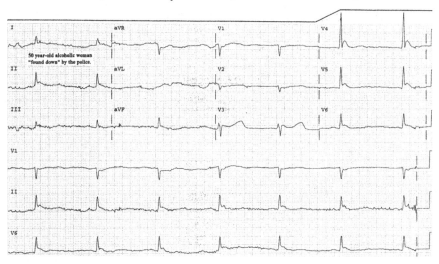

The J wave really should be called an upside down J wave, because that's what it looks like. You can see it clearly in leads V_4 and V_5. If you have difficulty making it out, get some glasses.

Central Nervous System Disorders

Severe central nervous system insults, such as large strokes or hemorrhagic bleeds, can lead to significant EKG abnormalities. The most common EKG finding is the presence of wide, deeply inverted T waves across the precordium. Note the example in figure 113.

Figure 113. EKG example of CNS insult: note the large deeply inverted T waves.

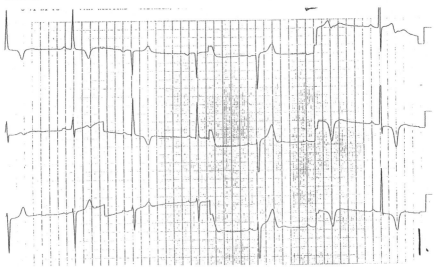

We don't really know why CNS insults cause such dramatic EKG changes, but we do know that you'll see them from time to time.

Ventricular Hypertrophy

Left ventricular hypertrophy (LVH) can cause an assortment of ST segment and T wave changes. Please be aware that inverted T waves and ST segment shifts can be a result of LVH alone and don't necessarily constitute ischemic heart disease. Symmetrically inverted T waves are more consistent with ischemia, whereas asymmetrically inverted T waves are generally because of LVH, but this isn't always the case. Note the example of LVH with secondary ST segment and T wave abnormalities seen in figure 114. We call this situation LVH with strain.

Figure 114. 12-lead of severe left ventricular hypertrophy: note the asymmetrically inverted T waves in V_4, V_5, and V_6. Note also increased QRS voltage.

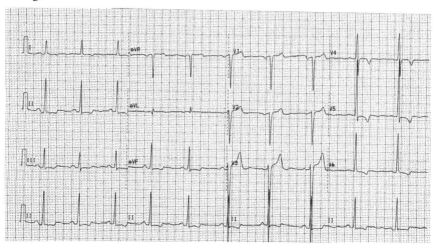

Digitalis Effect

Digitalis, a drug commonly used in the past, in patients with congestive heart failure, can have multiple effects on the EKG. The most common effect is that of **ST segment depression**. The ST segment looks like someone placed his or her finger on the ST segment and pulled it down as noted in figure 115. Other dig effects include arrhythmias, particularly **paroxysmal atrial tachycardia**.

Dig toxicity can occur despite a laboratory measurement confirming that it is within a "normal" serum dig range. So if your patient has an EKG finding consistent with digitalis toxicity and the laboratory reports a "normal" serum dig level, ignore the level and go with the EKG.

Figure 115. EKG showing digitalis effect. Note the pulled-down ST segments and the premature atrial contractions.

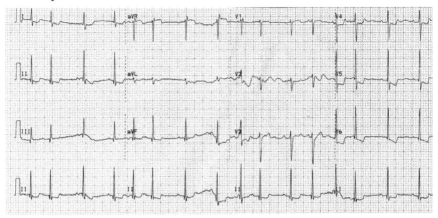

See how the ST segment in the lateral precordial leads looks as though someone took a finger and pulled it down.

There, of course, are many other miscellaneous and esoteric EKGs we could show you, but we want to keep this practical. If you have any further interest in a particular subject, you can look it up elsewhere.

CHAPTER 10: COMPLEX EKGS

When your car won't start, the best you can hope for is that something simple has happened to cause it to fail. Your best bet is that you didn't put gas in it, or maybe you left the lights on and the battery is dead. If you are like us, you won't be that lucky. More than likely, the repair will be involved and costly. Things aren't always simple—despite our wishing they were. Interpreting EKGs is similar to figuring out why a car won't start. There can be a simple reading on a fairly normal one, or a complex explanation of a difficult one. A normal EKG is easy to interpret. An abnormal EKG can have a single abnormality or multiple abnormalities. We want to help you with the process of rendering an opinion on EKGs that are abnormal in a complicated way. You are going to have to do it, so let's practice a little.

An EKG that is stone-cold normal is no challenge for even a marginally educated EKG interpreter. The reader of a normal EKG can even sound smart in the process of telling someone that the EKG is normal. For example the interpreter can say, "This patient has a normal sinus rhythm at a rate of 80 beats per minute with no sinus arrhythmia or premature atrial complexes. The QRS electrical vector calculates to plus 60 degrees, plus/minus five degrees. The PR interval is normal at 140 milliseconds. The QT interval calculates to 420 milliseconds, which is normal for the heart rate and the …" This could go on forever. Of course, the interpreter could just say that the patient has a normal EKG. That last approach might be a little brief and to the point, but it would be true.

The easier to read EKGs are those that have only one abnormality. For example, an EKG showing only a first-degree AV block is easy to interpret. You look at it and see that everything looks fine except the PR interval is longer than 200 milliseconds. With nothing else but a first-degree AV block being wrong with it, you can present it to your attending physician as an EKG with a normal sinus rhythm with a first-degree AV block with everything else being normal. You wouldn't actually say, "Everything else is normal." You are going to have to go into more detail, such as mentioning that the QRS axis is normal and that there are no abnormal Q waves or ST segment or T wave abnormalities.

An EKG showing four millimeters of ST segment elevation in leads II, III, and AVF would alert you to the diagnosis of an acute inferior infarct. An infarct can occasionally occur in a singular fashion, meaning that the infarct occurs in isolation with no other abnormality. Note that we said "occasionally occur," not commonly. So don't get used to looking for isolated abnormalities on EKGs. If you do, you will almost certainly miss some other important findings. Although isolated abnormalities can occur on some EKGs, more commonly you will find that as one thing goes wrong, so goes many.

Given that the law of parsimony (also known as Occam's razor) rarely applies to EKGs, it would be useful to you, as a young EKG reader, to know how to diagnose and present abnormalities found on complex EKGs. It also would be helpful for you to be familiar with what abnormalities commonly occur together. If you go in search of something, you need to know what you are searching for before you go out on the trail to find it. To help you, we would like to teach you **that if you see this, then we want you to think of and look for that**. Let's look at how to organize your analysis of complicated EKGs first—this will be easy and has really already been presented, but it bears reviewing.

If you look at the beginning of this book, you will see how we presented a perfect sequence of analysis that we suggested you follow when reading EKGs. If you follow this sequence in its entirety and render your opinion verbally, the poor soul listening to your diatribe will likely prefer to be shot. Nevertheless, you'll at least have comfort in knowing that you didn't miss much that was wrong with the EKG. The difficulty for you, the reader, won't be in following the sequence we have outlined; rather, it will be in the conclusions you draw after you have read the EKG. Also, you will find that your style of presentation of your overall impression once you have looked at and read the EKG will need to be practiced and polished. It is here that things can become tricky. There's not only one correct way to present the information you have gleaned from interpreting a specific EKG—and we won't try to persuade you that there is. We would encourage you to use some common sense, though. Let us illustrate this metaphorically.

Suppose you came home and looked in the bathroom mirror and happened to notice that your hair was on fire. You see the fire, but the reason you came into the bathroom is because you needed to go to the bathroom. What would you do first? Would you go to the bathroom, or would you put out the fire on your head?

Look at the EKG in figure 116. When you look at that EKG, what is the first thing you notice? If you said an acute inferior infarct, you're right. Keep looking—what else do you see? You have to look carefully to tell. Look in V_1 and see the P wave. Do you notice the terminal portion of the P wave is inverted and wide indicative of left atrial enlargement?

Figure 116. 12-lead example of an inferior infarct and LAE.

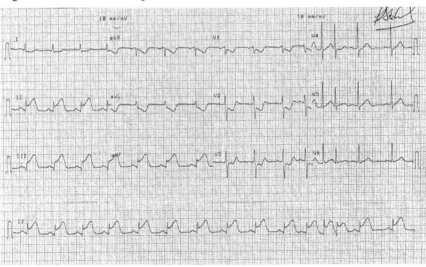

If you were asked to tell someone what this EKG shows, you would probably start with the infarct part first, as it is more important than the LAE. The take home from this little illustration is that you should mention the most important thing happening to the patient first, but don't fail to be complete. The checklist we gave you earlier should serve as a guide to make sure you don't overlook anything, but common sense should prevail when you present your findings.

Look at the tracing in figure 117. This one has several things going on. You'll have to be organized to get all the detail. See how many abnormalities you can find and write them down before we give you the answers.

Figure 117. Unknown complex 12-lead example.

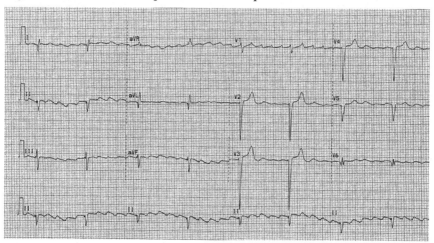

Now that you've had a chance to familiarize yourself with the above example, let's start with what is immediately apparent as abnormal. Notice the rate. What is it? It's less than sixty beats per minute (actually forty-eight). What is the rhythm? Is it sinus, or some other? It's atrial flutter with very slow AV conduction. If you look carefully, you'll see that it takes about five or six flutter waves to get through the AV node to cause a QRS complex. Now, what is the axis? It's not normal. It's extreme, extreme right-axis deviation—pointing directly toward AVR. When you see this type of axis, you need to think of a left posterior fascicular block, right ventricular hypertophy, and a lateral wall infarct. Look, you see Q waves in I, AVL, and V_4, V_5, and V_6. This is truly a complicated EKG. We would summarize it as atrial flutter with some pathologic degree of AV block, large anterolateral myocardial infarction with extreme right axis suggestive of a left posterior fascicular block, as well. We know this was a challenge, but we wanted to help you learn how to organize your thoughts.

Now, let's look, in no particular order, at what maladies often occur in concert with each other. We won't come close to covering them all, but it should be worth your while to review the following pairings that we have chosen.

One of the more common associations you'll come across is that of left ventricular hypertrophy occurring coincidentally with LAE. There is a physiological reason for this that you might want to know, so we'll mention it. As untreated hypertension occurs, the left ventricle is forced to work harder than usual to overcome the abnormally elevated peripheral vascular resistance. Over time, the left ventricle adapts to its increased workload by thickening. In a way, it's similar to exercising your skeletal muscles and witnessing the hypertophy that accompanies it. Unfortunately, as the left ventricle thickens, it becomes less compliant. That is to say, it loses its elasticity. It's the job of the left atrium to contract and force blood into the left ventricle to facilitate its filling. You can then imagine that as the left ventricle becomes less compliant, or stiffer, the left atrium will have to squeeze harder to do its job. The left atrium will adapt to its increased workload by enlarging. See figure 118.

Figure 118. 12-lead example of LVH and LAE.

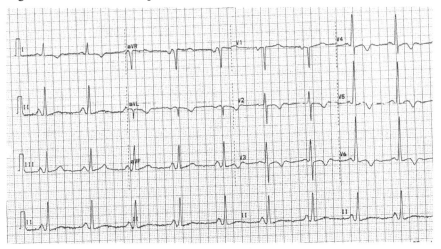

If LAE occurs with left ventricular enlargement, then right atrial enlargement occurs with RVE. The EKG in figure 119 illustrates many things. At first glance, you'll notice in lead I that its baseline is wandering. The reason it wanders is because this patient was short of breath during the EKG recording. Lead I also shows the aforementioned Schamroth sign, which suggests right ventricular enlargement that accompanies chronic obstructive pulmonary disease. All this information should alert you to the possibility of RAE. Now look in leads II, III, and AVF, and you'll see peaked P waves.

Figure 119. 12-lead example of Schamroth'sign and RAE.

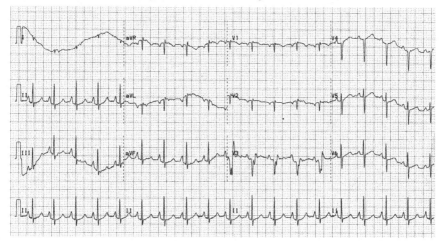

If you ever had the opportunity to play football, then you know that if you were asked to block someone on the opposing team and were successful, then you shouldn't be satisfied with blocking just one guy. You should try to block as many people as possible! Electrical blocks of the conduction system in the heart behave in a manner similar to what is expected of football players. Frequently, electrical or conduction blocks occur only in one circuit. Other times they occur in multiple areas, as the example in figure 120 illustrates. This EKG was obtained on a patient who kept having syncope (passing out). Note the RSR prime configuration in lead V_1. Also note the deep S wave in lead I. The QRS duration is just short of 120 milliseconds. Based on this, you can correctly state that the patient has an incomplete right bundle branch block. Keep looking though. What else do you notice? The PR interval is just inside of normal at 190 milliseconds, so no first-degree AV block is present. The EKG does have extreme right axis deviation, however. This extreme right axis deviation tells you that the patient also has a left posterior fascicular block. No wonder this patient kept passing out. He was living off a sick right bundle and a functioning left anterior fascicle only, which likely also occasionally failed, resulting in prolonged episodes of no heartbeat for this patient. No need to puzzle anymore about why this patient was having trouble.

Figure 120. 12-lead example of an incomplete RBBB and LPFB.

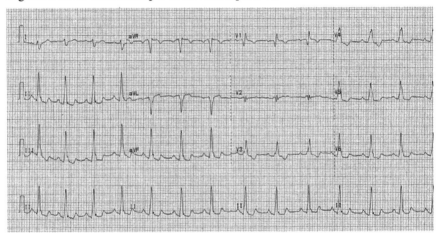

So blocks tend to occur together, especially right bundle branch blocks with left anterior or left posterior fascicular blocks. Left bundle branch blocks occur with first-degree AV blocks and more high-grade AV blocks. The ultimate block, short of no heartbeat at all, is a left bundle branch block with complete heart block, as shown in figure 121.

Figure 121. 12-lead example of LBBB and complete heart block.

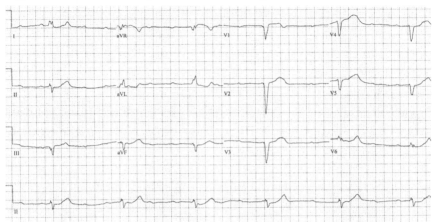

Although we don't show any examples here, be aware that electrolyte abnormalities often occur together. For example, hypokalemia and hypomagnesemia often occur at the same time in the same patient. The reason for this is usually self-evident—the alcoholic patient who vomits and fails to eat properly. From a clinical standpoint, especially if you are a physician, it's important to keep this in mind when treating patients.

Now let's look at just a couple more examples to round out your education. Look at the EKG in figure 122. Just look at the EKG as a stand-alone item with no clinical information. What do you notice first? Do you see the global ST segment elevation? Yes, you do. So, what is your diagnosis? We hope you said pericarditis. Good, you're getting it, but you're actually wrong. This EKG, even though it looks like pericarditis, isn't. Look closely. Do you see concomitant PR segment depression? Would it help if we told you the EKG was obtained on a young black male?

Figure 122. 12-lead example of early repolarization.

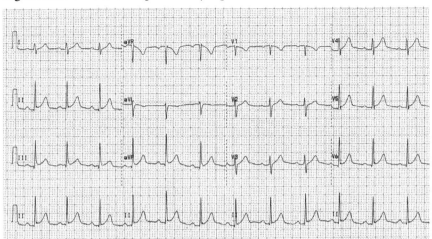

Yes, this is a perfect example of the early repolarization phenomenon. It's a normal variant in young black men. Use the history to help you, if you're lucky enough to get it.

This last example (fig. 123) is useful in teaching you the importance of looking closely and having an open mind. First, take a long and careful look at it. Jot down the rate and the rhythm. We can't calculate the axis, because this is a continuous three-lead rhythm strip.

Figure 123. 3-lead example of an unknown EKG.

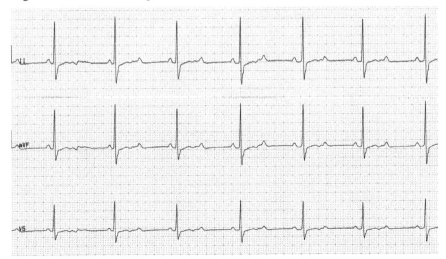

At first glance, the rate on this example appears to be about 40 beats per minute. At least that is the ventricular rate. What is the atrial rate? Is it 40 as well? Look closely at the T waves. Do you see P waves hidden at the end of the T waves, deforming them just a little? The atrial rate in this example is actually around 80 beats per minute. So in this example, the atrial rate and the ventricular rate don't match. What is happening here is that there is 2-to-1 AV conduction, where every other P wave is blocked. This is a great example of normal sinus rhythm with a 2-to-1 AV block. Always search the T waves for hidden P waves. In this case, the hidden P wave gives the appearance of a prominent U wave. Can you see how easily you can draw an inaccurate conclusion if you don't take the time to look carefully at everything in a systematic manner?

There is no end to how complex EKGs can be. There is an end, however, to the text of this book, and it's occurring here. Now, proceed to the final chapter to test yourself some more.

CHAPTER 11: CLINICAL CASES AND EKG PEARLS

The best way to learn EKGS is to look at many different cases!

Having read and learned the preceding material, you're now ready to test your knowledge. We believe that the best approach to cement your knowledge is to try out your new skills on various practice tracings. These EKG examples have been carefully selected to illustrate clinical pearls and to confirm that you have learned something useful about common and important EKG abnormalities. Clinical scenarios are included to help you put the EKG into a "real-world" context. We are convinced that doing so will make you much more likely to remember what is important. We have found, through our experience with working with Boneheads, that disjointed facts are quickly forgotten if there is no practical application for the information. So venture forth, read the clinical scenarios, review the EKGs, and answer the questions as they are posed. Maintain a sense of levity as you muddle your way through these examples.

1. The tracing shown in figure 124 was performed on a twenty-one-year-old white male who presented to our office complaining of substernal chest pain. The patient had a viral illness two weeks prior from which he predominantly recovered; however, three days ago he developed discomfort in the center of his chest. The sensation was described as sharp and catchy in nature. He also developed a low-grade fever and had difficulty lying supine because of the discomfort.

Figure 124.

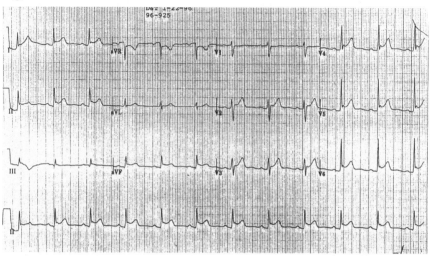

Review the tracing above and answer the following question:
After obtaining this EKG on this patient, what would your next
course of action be?

    a. Reassure the patient that his EKG is absolutely normal
        and that his symptoms are completely fabricated.

    b. Refer him to an orthopedic surgeon for removal of his
        sternum.

    c. Give him thrombolytic therapy and take him to the cath
        lab for urgent cardiac catheterization. (One of the authors
        on the cardiology boards chose this! *Don't do this!*)

    d. Administer relatively high-dose nonsteroidal-anti-
        inflammatory drugs, and/or colchicine for pericarditis.

If you answered D, you're correct. This patient has pericarditis.
Note the global ST segment elevation and the P-R segment
depression. Also note that AVR, once again, is the oddball lead
where the ST and P-R segment changes are reversed. Most often,
pericarditis is treated with nonsteroidal-anti-inflammatory
drugs. Recalcitrant cases can be treated with steroids, but
we like to avoid these because this might lead to relapsing
pericarditis. You would never want to give a patient with

pericarditis thrombolytic agents or blood thinners because this could result in a hemorrhagic pericardial effusion that might lead to tamponade and patient death. Of course, now that you have completed this book, you wouldn't make that mistake.

2. The EKG in figure 125 is that of a sixty-year-old white male who presented to the hospital with three hours of substernal chest pain. He smokes and has diabetes mellitus and hyperlipidemia. He had some associated diaphoresis (sweating) and shortness of breath with the onset of the chest pain.

Figure 125.

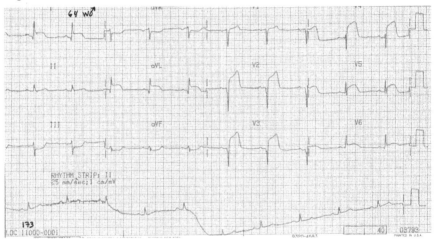

Now attempt to answer the following question:
As a Bonehead doctor when presented with this EKG, your next step would be to:

 a. Ask the nurse to obtain another tracing because this EKG clearly couldn't be from this patient.

 b. Check the patient's cholesterol level.

 c. Pat the patient on the back and tell him that you're an orthopedic surgeon and that you don't know anything about EKGs.

 d. Give him aspirin, IV nitroglycerin, and heparin (a blood thinner) and call the cardiologist pronto.

If you answered D, you're correct. This patient does have an acute anterolateral wall myocardial infarction. Notice that there is marked ST segment elevation across the precordial leads. The configuration of the ST segment elevation is concave upward. Another way to word this is that it is convex. These are called **tombstone** ST segments. They represent an acute transmural myocardial infarction which will require immediate attention. Notice that the ST segment elevation is limited primarily to the anterior and lateral leads. The inferior leads are spared, and even reciprocally depressed. There isn't global ST segment elevation as noted in acute pericarditis.

3. The EKG in figure 126 belongs to a forty-eight-year-old black male who presented with lower extremity edema and decreased urine output over the past week or so.

Figure 126.

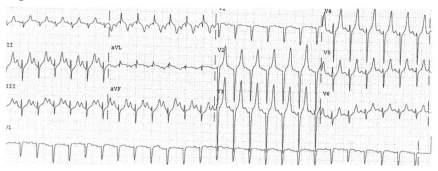

Please answer the following question.
When presented with this EKG, the next appropriate step for the Bonehead physician is to:

a. Refer for outpatient consultation with a nephrologist.
b. Refer for outpatient consultation with a vascular medicine physician for evaluation of edema.
c. Administer a high concentration of potassium chloride solution intravenously.

    d. Move this patient immediately to the Intensive Care Unit and prepare to treat him for marked hyperkalemia.

Again, if you answered D, you are correct (and since an astute reader such as yourself is sure you're seeing the pattern here, we won't mention this again). The EKG in this particular example belonged to a patient who had a potassium level of 10 mg/dl (normal 4.5). Had his potassium level not been corrected immediately, he would have been unavailable for any future mud-wrestling activities. Hyperkalemia that causes EKG changes of a similar nature to this requires immediate attention to prevent ventricular fibrillation. Note the mildly widened QRS complexes and the peaked and pinched T waves. Patients with less marked elevations of potassium might present only with peaked T waves.

4. Please review the EKG in figure 127. This tracing belonged to a twenty-two-year-old female who had been complaining of palpitations for years. She had never been taken seriously by her physician. Now, try to answer the following question.

Figure 127.

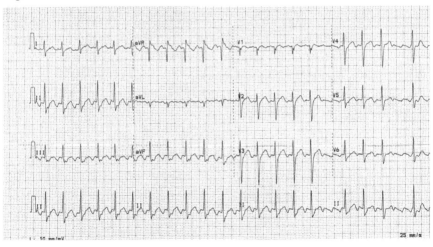

As a Bonehead physician, after obtaining this tracing you would:

a. Tell the patient and her family that she really needs to have her panic disorder treated and that you would like to refer her to a psychiatrist.

b. Place a 24-hour Holter monitor and see her back in clinic in a few weeks.

c. Tell her that her heart rate is too slow and implant a permanent pacemaker.

d. Perform carotid sinus massage and/or prepare to electrically cardiovert her.

The tracing in figure 127 demonstrates supraventricular tachycardia at a rapid rate. Notice that the QRS complexes are narrow and also obvious is that there is a sawtooth pattern seen best in the inferior leads. The sawtooth pattern is a clue that this is atrial flutter with 2-to-1 conduction. On the tracing below, the patient was given adenosine. Adenosine will slow AV conduction transiently. See the emergence of the classical atrial flutter pattern when the adenosine is administered. The clue to atrial flutter is that the ventricular response rate is 150 beats a minute, which generally runs at about 300 beats per minute. You don't normally electrically cardiovert atrial flutter or supraventricular tachycardia unless the patient is hemodynamically unstable— that is, unless you are a masochist. See also in the subsequent example that follows the immediate strip below of what happens when adenosine is given (see figs. 128 and 129).

Figure 128. Rhythm strip before adenosine.

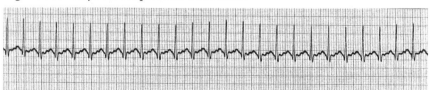

Figure 129. After adenosine.

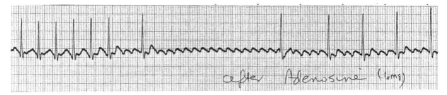

5. The EKG in figure 130 belongs to a seventeen-year-old track star at a local high school. He was checking his pulse one day while he was daydreaming during calculus class. At that time, he noted that his heart skipped a beat; as you can guess, he ran to his family doctor, who happens to be you, and had this EKG rhythm strip performed.

Figure 130.

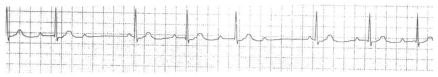

Answer the following questions relative to the EKG rhythm strip:

When presented with this rhythm strip, you would:

    a. Immediately admit him to the hospital for diagnostic cardiac catheterization and pacemaker implantation.

    b. Ask him to stop abusing sleeping medicine.

    c. Refer him to a cardiac transplant center for cardiac transplant.

    d. Reassure him that this particular heart rhythm is often normal for a well-trained athlete.

In the tracing in figure 130, please note that there are skipped beats. You will notice that there is a pattern of grouped beating. Notice also that the P-R interval progressively lengthens, getting gradually longer and longer, until finally a QRS complex is dropped. Immediately after the dropped beat, the PR interval shortens back to a normal length. The process will repeat itself following this same format. This is the hallmark of Mobitz I second-degree AV block. Recall this is also called Wenckebach block. This is a "normal heart rhythm" in many people. Its presence rarely indicates significant cardiac pathology.

6. The EKG in figure 131 was obtained on a seventy-two-year-old black female with long-standing hypertension. The patient had no complaints. She was in for a routine physical.

Figure 131.

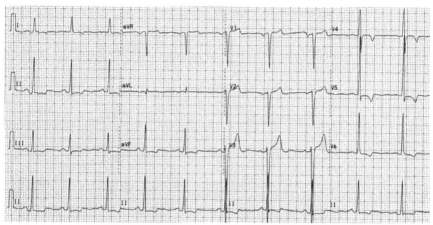

Upon being presented with this EKG, you would advise the patient the following:

a. You expected payment when services are rendered.
b. Hypertension is really not that bad and that if she practices meditation, it might go away.
c. She is obviously not getting enough salt in her diet.
d. An echocardiogram might be in order to assess the size of her left atrium and left ventricle.

This patient has evidence of severe left ventricular and left atrial enlargement. For the LAE component, look in lead V$_1$ and notice that the terminal portion of the P wave is deeply inverted and wide. This is the hallmark of LAE that we want you to remember. Also note the increased QRS voltage and the secondary ST-T wave changes; this is a marker for left ventricular hypertrophy. Add up the deepest S wave in V_1 or V_2, to the tallest R wave in V_5 or V_6, and you'll calculate that it's much greater than 35 mm. If this is the case, the patient likely has LVH. In this particular example, there are also secondary changes, which help to support the diagnosis of LVH. The clinical pearl here is that hypertension is deadly and needs to be treated to prevent secondary complications, which include congestive heart failure, kidney disease, and stroke.

7. The rhythm strip in figure 132 was obtained on a college student who had a Super Bowl party. At the party, he consumed quite a bit of alcohol. He couldn't quite remember what he did Sunday night; however, Monday morning he did make it to class, but noticed his heart beating irregularly. He got scared and presented with this EKG.

Figure 132.

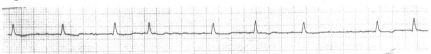

Upon reviewing this EKG, you advise this college graduate student to:

   a. Drink a different brand of beer.
   b. Switch from beer to liquor only.
   c. Invite you to his next party.
   d. Avoid excessive alcohol now and in the future because he has holiday heart syndrome.

This patient's rhythm strip reveals atrial fibrillation. Note that there's a lack of discernible P wave activity and that the QRSs occur in an irregularly irregular fashion. This is characteristic of atrial fibrillation. For your information, holiday heart syndrome is a clinical problem that occurs frequently in all demographics, not just college students. It is episodic atrial fibrillation following a drinking binge (which, no doubt, you've never done). Atrial fibrillation generally resolves shortly thereafter but might require medical therapy or cardioversion. Most youngsters on no medication would have a much faster heart rate than the example above shows.

8. The EKG in figure 133 was obtained on a patient with chronic obstructive pulmonary disease. The patient had been a long-time smoker and was exposed to asbestos. He presented with dyspnea. This EKG was obtained in the emergency room as he was being admitted for an acute bronchitis episode.

Figure 133.

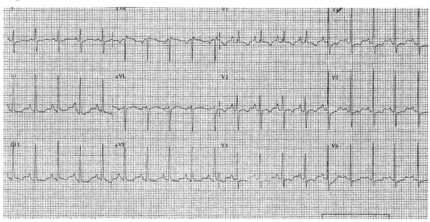

Upon obtaining this EKG, you would:

a. Assume that his blue-appearing fingertips were because of cyanide poisoning and place him in a hyperbaric oxygen chamber.

b. Assume that his barrel-shaped chest was because of the fact that he was an Olympic swimmer as a youngster.

c. Assume that the edema in his lower extremities was because of the long bus ride over to the hospital.

   d. Listen to his lungs and expect to hear expiratory wheezing.

This EKG reveals an incomplete right bundle branch block and RAE. Notice the RSR configuration in lead V_1. Also note the peaked P waves in the inferior leads. This is evidence of RAE, which is commonly seen in patients with underlying pulmonary disease.

9. What does the EKG in figure 134 suggest to you?

Figure 134.

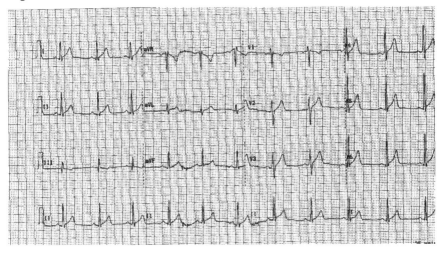

   a. Pericarditis
   b. Acute myocardial infarction
   c. LVH with repolarization changes
   d. Normal variant in a young black male

D is correct. This EKG illustrates how important it is to have clinical information to go along with the tracing you're trying to interpret. If the patient had sharp chest pain and a fever, then pericarditis would have been suggested. Close examination, however, would have failed to reveal PR segment depression, also seen in pericarditis. Early repolarization changes with the appearance of ST segment elevation are a normal finding in some patients, particularly young black men.

10. The EKG in figure 135 was obtained on an apparently healthy twenty-year-old college tennis player as part of a preparticipation physical exam. What is wrong with this athlete?

Figure 135.

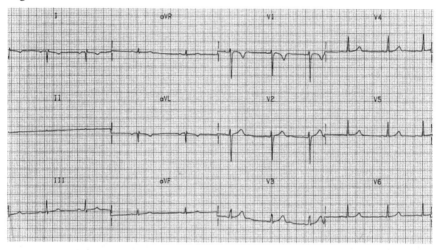

    a. He has dextrocardia.

    b. He had a high-lateral infarct causing Q waves in I and AVL.

    c. He has an ectopic atrial focus causing upright P waves in AVR.

    d. The EKG technician misplaced the leads.

Again, D is correct. The clue that the technician is at fault is that the P waves are upright in AVR. We know this can't be the case if the rhythm is sinus. Sinus rhythm dictates that the P wave axis be oriented inferiorly. So, normally, the P wave axis is directed away from AVR, resulting in inverted P waves in that lead. We can explain the extreme right axis and Q waves in I and AVL as the result of inattentive and careless work on the part of the technician.

That should do it for the practice questions. You might have noticed that we used them as a springboard for discussion of important subjects. We hope that will help you remember what we believe is important.

When speaking of EKGs, the subject matter is vast, and the potential permutations and combinations of abnormalities are almost infinite, so we can't cover it all. Actually we could, but you wouldn't want to take the time to read a book several thousand pages long. We hope you've learned as much as you hoped was possible from the text and the examples that we carefully chose for your edification.

We leave you with this advice: be informed, be interested, be observant, be organized, be succinct, and be humble. But most importantly of all, if your ambition is to become a physician, be compassionate. Compassion toward those who suffer is sometimes hard to learn and all too easy to forget when you are tired, hungry, and frustrated.

Thank you for allowing us to impart some of our knowledge into your Bonehead brains!

John R. Hicks, MD
Floyd W. Burke, MD

Printed in the United States
By Bookmasters